Anne Hiller Scott, PhD, OTR, FAOTA
Editor

New Frontiers in Psychosocial Occupational Therapy

New Frontiers in Psychosocial Occupational Therapy has been co-published simultaneously as *Occupational Therapy in Mental Health,* Volume 14, Numbers 1/2 1998.

Pre-publication REVIEWS, COMMENTARIES, EVALUATIONS . . .

"**N**ew Frontiers in Psychosocial Occupational Therapy speaks a clear message about mental health practice in occupational therapy–shattering old visions of practice to insights about empowerment and advocacy. Now we have solid advice which for the first time offers hope and methods to reverse a downward spiral. This publication demonstrates the process of reclaiming our destiny as mental health practitioners with consumers and students the guides."

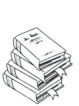

Sharan L. Schwartzberg, EdD, OTR, FAOTA
Professor and Chair
Boston School of Occupational Therapy
Tufts University

D0081992

"**D**rawing on the expertise of veteran clinicians and educators, the perspectives of consumers, and the vision and spontaneity of students on their first fieldwork, Scott has gathered inspiring and practical articles for this small volume. Practitioners will find models and precedents for 'breaking out of the box' and academic and clinical educators will find easily-implemented strategies for classroom and fieldwork. The articles are varied in their authorship, emphasis, and content. This is a valuable guide for occupational therapy practitioners who seek to create a practice for tomorrow."

Mary Beth Early, MS, OTR/L
Professor
La Guardia Community College
Long Island City
New York

"*New Frontiers in Psychosocial Therapy* is a call to arms for occupational therapists. This book identifies the many challenges of mental health practice in general while delineating specific concerns for occupational therapists. However, the real value of this book lies in its solutions. Some important issues addressed include finding meaning and purpose in your work, increased awareness of legislation and mental health systems, use of technology, and the need to develop community-based, empowerment models of practice. Different perspectives and multiple examples provide practical approaches so that occupational therapists can address today's challenges with a sense of direction and confidence. The inclusion of the voice of consumers and occupational therapy students contributes an important but commonly neglected viewpoint."

Catana Brown, MA, OTR
Assistant Professor
University of Kansas
Medical Center

"**M**y immediate reaction, in the 'Introduction,' was that–this needs to go to students in healthcare administration as well as to students of occupational therapy. Susan Fine's chapter evokes the image of someone in the pulpit admonishing the greed soaked healthcare delivery system. It expresses the emotions bubbling up to the surface from therapists inundated with change. It assures therapists that they are not alone in their frustrations with this rapid change.

The consumer stories are so gripping. Explanation of the Americans with Disabilities Act (ADA) helps students understand the subtleties and ambiguities of applying the ADA in mental health. Ideas of empowerment, such as asking consumers/clients to write their own progress notes, prepare them to fit in the culture in which individuals are constantly asked to take more and more responsibility for themselves. Suggestions for thinking about sexual harassment will prepare fieldwork students and therapists for the all too common situation of patient 'come-ons.'

The chapter on the Internet is simple enough for someone never before exposed to Internet use.

A thorough description takes the reader through an easily understandable progression to demonstrate how computers can strengthen mental health occupational therapy treatment.

Occupational therapy educators will immediately want to implement ideas presented. Fieldwork coordinators will find new ways of assisting students to develop insight about their treatment approaches. This is the book for this age in healthcare."

Margaret Drake, PhD, OTR/L, ATR-BC, FAOTA
Associate Professor
University of Mississippi
Medical Center
School of Health Related Professions
Department of Occupational Therapy

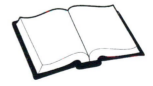

The Haworth Press, Inc.

New Frontiers in Psychosocial Occupational Therapy

New Frontiers in Psychosocial Occupational Therapy has been co-published simultaneously as *Occupational Therapy in Mental Health*, Volume 14, Numbers 1/2 1998.

The *Occupational Therapy in Mental Health* Monographs/"Separates"

Psychiatric Occupational Therapy in the Army, edited by LTC Paul D. Ellsworth and Diane Gibson

Occupational Therapy with Borderline Patients, edited by Diane Gibson

SCORE: Solving Community Obstacles and Restoring Employment, by Lynn Wechsler Kramer

Short-Term Treatment in Occupational Therapy, edited by Diane Gibson and Kathy Kaplan

Philosophical and Historical Roots of Occupational Therapy, edited by Karen Diasio Serrett

The Evaluation and Treatment of Eating Disorders, edited by Diane Gibson

Treatment of the Chronic Schizophrenic Patient, edited by Diane Gibson

Evaluation and Treatment of Adolescents and Children, edited by Diane Gibson

The Development of Standardized Clinical Evaluations in Mental Health edited by Claudia Kay Allen, Principal Investigator: Noomi Katz, and Commentator: Janice P. Burke

Treatment of Substance Abuse: Psychosocial Occupational Therapy Approaches, edited by Diane Gibson

Group Process and Structure in Psychosocial Occupational Therapy, edited by Diane Gibson

Instrument Development in Occupational Therapy, edited by Janet Hawkins Watts and Chestina Brollier

Group Protocols: A Psychosocial Compendium, edited by Susan Haiman

Student Recruitment in Psychosocial Occupational Therapy: Intergenerational Approaches, edited by Susan Haiman

Evaluation and Treatment of the Psychogeriatric Patient, edited by Diane Gibson

New Frontiers in Psychosocial Occupational Therapy, edited by Anne Hiller Scott

These books were published simultaneously as special thematic issues of *Occupational Therapy in Mental Health* and are available bound separately. Visit Haworth's website at http://www.haworthpressinc.com to search our online catalog for complete tables of contents and ordering information for these and other publications. Or call 1-800-HAWORTH (outside US/Canada: 607-722-5857), Fax: 1-800-895-0582 (outside US/Canada: 607-771-0012), or e-mail getinfo@ haworthpressinc.com

New Frontiers in Psychosocial Occupational Therapy

Anne Hiller Scott, PhD, OTR, FAOTA
Editor

New Frontiers in Psychosocial Occupational Therapy has been co-published simultaneously as *Occupational Therapy in Mental Health*, Volume 14, Numbers 1/2 1998.

The Haworth Press, Inc.
New York • London

New Frontiers in Psychosocial Occupational Therapy has been co-published simultaneously as *Occupational Therapy in Mental Health*™, Volume 14, Numbers 1/2 1998.

The Haworth Press, Inc., 10 Alice Street, Binghamton, NY 13904-1580 USA

Cover design by Thomas J. Mayshock Jr.

Library of Congress Cataloging-in-Publication Data

New frontiers in psychosocial occupational therapy / Anne Hiller Scott, editor.
      p. cm.
      "New frontiers in psychosocial occupational therapy has been co-published as Occupational therapy in mental health, Volume 14, numbers 1/2 1998."
      Includes bibliographical references and index.
      ISBN 0-7890-0652-9 (alk. paper)
      1. Occupational therapy–Practice–United States. I. Scott, Anne Hiller.
RC487.N49 1998
362.2'0425–dc21
                                           98-36240
                                                CIP

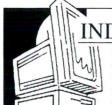

INDEXING & ABSTRACTING

Contributions to this publication are selectively indexed or abstracted in print, electronic, online, or CD-ROM version(s) of the reference tools and information services listed below. This list is current as of the copyright date of this publication. See the end of this section for additional notes.

- *Abstracts in Social Gerontology: Current Literature on Aging,* National Council on the Aging, Library, 409 Third Street SW, 2nd Floor, Washington, DC 20024

- *Alzheimer's Disease Education & Referral Center (ADEAR),* Combined Health Information Database (CHID), P.O. Box 8250, Silver Spring, MD 20907-8250

- *CINAHL (Cumulative Index to Nursing & Allied Health Literature), in print, also on CD-ROM from CD PLUS, EBSCO, and SilverPlatter, and online from CDP Online (formerly BRS), Data-Star, and PaperChase. (Support materials include Subject Heading List, Database Search Guide, and instructional video.),* CINAHL Information Systems, P.O. Box 871/1509 Wilson Terrace, Glendale, CA 91209-0871

- *CNPIEC Reference Guide: Chinese National Directory of Foreign Periodicals,* P.O. Box 88, Beijing, People's Republic of China

- *Developmental Medicine & Child Neurology,* Mac Keith Press, 526-529 High Holborn House, 52-54 High Holborn, London WC1V 6RL, England

- *Exceptional Child Education Resources (ECER), (CD/ROM from SilverPlatter and hard copy),* The Council for Exceptional Children, 1920 Association Drive, Reston, VA 20191-1589

- *EMBASE/Excerpta Medica Secondary Publishing Division,* Elsevier Science Inc., Secondary Publishing Division, 655 Avenue of the Americas, New York, NY 10010

- *Family Studies Database (online and CD/ROM),* National Information Services Corporation, 306 East Baltimore Pike, 2nd Floor, Media, PA 19063

(continued)

- *INTERNET ACCESS (& additional networks) Bulletin Board for Libraries ("BUBL") coverage of information resources on INTERNET, JANET, and other networks.*
  - <URL:http://bubl.ac.uk/>
  - The new locations will be found under <URL:http://bubl.ac.uk/link/>.
  - Any existing BUBL users who have problems finding information on the new service should contact the BUBL help line by sending e-mail to <bubl@bubl.ac.uk>.

  The Andersonian Library, Curran Building, 101 St. James Road, Glasgow G4 0NS, Scotland

- *Mental Health Abstracts (online through DIALOG),* IFI/Plenum Data Company, 3202 Kirkwood Highway, Wilmington, DE 19808

- *Occupational Therapy Database (OTDBASE),* 3485 Point Grey Road, Vancouver, BC V6R 1A6, Canada

- *Occupational Therapy Index,* British Library Medical Information Service, Boston Spa, Wetherby, West Yorkshire, LS23 7BQ, United Kingdom

- *OT BibSys,* American Occupational Therapy Foundation, P.O. Box 31220, Rockville, MD 20824-1220

- *PASCAL, c/o Institute de L'Information Scientifique et Technique. Cross-disciplinary electronic database covering the fields of science, technology & medicine. Also available on CD-ROM, and can generate customized retrospective searches. For information: INIST, Customer Desk, 2, allee du Parc de Brabois, F-54514 Vandoeuvre Cedex, France; http//www.inist.fr,* INIST/CNRS-Service Gestion des Documents Primaires, 2, allee du Parc de Brabois, F-54514 Vandoeuvre-les-Nancy, Cedex, France

- *Psychiatric Rehabilitation Journal,* 930 Commonwealth Avenue, Boston, MA 02215

- *Social Work Abstracts,* National Association of Social Workers, 750 First Street NW, 8th Floor, Washington, DC 20002

- *Sport Search,* Sport Information Resource Center, 1600 James Naismith Drive, Suite 107, Gloucester, Ontario K1B 5N4, Canada

(continued)

SPECIAL BIBLIOGRAPHIC NOTES

related to special journal issues (separates)
and indexing/abstracting

☐ indexing/abstracting services in this list will also cover material in any "separate" that is co-published simultaneously with Haworth's special thematic journal issue or DocuSerial. Indexing/abstracting usually covers material at the article/chapter level.

☐ monographic co-editions are intended for either non-subscribers or libraries which intend to purchase a second copy for their circulating collections.

☐ monographic co-editions are reported to all jobbers/wholesalers/approval plans. The source journal is listed as the "series" to assist the prevention of duplicate purchasing in the same manner utilized for books-in-series.

☐ to facilitate user/access services all indexing/abstracting services are encouraged to utilize the co-indexing entry note indicated at the bottom of the first page of each article/chapter/contribution.

☐ this is intended to assist a library user of any reference tool (whether print, electronic, online, or CD-ROM) to locate the monographic version if the library has purchased this version but not a subscription to the source journal.

☐ individual articles/chapters in any Haworth publication are also available through the Haworth Document Delivery Service (HDDS).

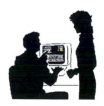

ALL HAWORTH BOOKS AND JOURNALS
ARE PRINTED ON CERTIFIED
ACID-FREE PAPER

New Frontiers in Psychosocial Occupational Therapy

CONTENTS

ABOUT THE EDITOR

Anne Hiller Scott, PhD, OTR, FAOTA, is Director of the Division of Occupational Therapy at Long Island University, Brooklyn Campus. She is a frequent presenter at international, national, and state venues, most recently presenting on the topics of working with consumers of mental health services, forming local and national networks of occupational therapists to promote mental health practice, and developing community-based health promotion programs. With over two decades' experience in practice and education, she has written numerous chapters and articles on occupational therapy in mental health and is a member of the national education honor society, Kappa Delta Pi, and a Fellow of the American Occupational Therapy Association. In addition, Dr. Scott has actively worked with the Metropolitan New York State District Occupational Therapy Association (MNYD of NYSOTA) Mental Health Task Force to promote mental health services for patients and clients in the community. Currently, she is developing an on-line web page, in conjunction with MNYD and the New Jersey Network on Wellness, that will serve as a directory for community-oriented, holistic interventions for occupational therapy practitioners and consumers.

Introduction:
New Frontiers in Mental Health

Anne Hiller Scott, PhD, OTR, FAOTA

The theme of this volume is *New Frontiers in Mental Health*. The *New Frontier* was part of the legacy of President John F. Kennedy, who during his administration set ambitious goals for the exploration of space. This period also witnessed the dawning of de-institutionalization ushered in by the Community Mental Health Centers Act of 1963. However, it was in fact, far easier to venture into the domain of outer space than to conquer "inner space" and the infinite reaches of the human mind. Although this ground-breaking legislation of the Kennedy era presaged a major realignment in the philosophy and treatment of the mentally ill, the reforms envisioned in the community mental health movement often failed to materialize for many of those in greatest need. Will the same be said of the current health care revolution?

Health care as we know it may not survive the organization of managed care. The prospects for occupational therapy in mental health in the twenty-first century are threatened. In this publication, we imagine an opportunity for new frontiers informed by our knowledge of the successes and failures of past paradigms. Visionary efforts are needed to direct us through to the new frontiers. Therapists must recognize opportunities for change to effectively define and deliver innovative practice in a new marketplace and to

[Haworth co-indexing entry note]: "Introduction: New Frontiers in Mental Health." Scott, Anne Hiller. Co-published simultaneously in *Occupational Therapy in Mental Health* (The Haworth Press, Inc.) Vol. 14, No. 1/2, 1998, pp. 1-6; and: *New Frontiers in Psychosocial Occupational Therapy* (ed: Anne Hiller Scott) The Haworth Press, Inc., 1998, pp. 1-6. Single or multiple copies of this article are available for a fee from The Haworth Document Delivery Service [1-800-342-9678, 9:00 a.m. - 5:00 p.m. (EST). E-mail address: getinfo@haworthpressinc.com].

1

assume leadership roles and partnerships with consumers and other professionals.

NEW FRONTIERS, PARTNERSHIPS AND PRACTICE OPPORTUNITIES

This book will focus on visions of new frontiers from many perspectives: practice, education, technology, organizational and societal change and local and state advocacy. Importantly, consumer perspectives are also represented. In the series of articles beginning with "Dialogue with Consumers" the views of consumers and mental health advocates will be presented. Part of our challenge is to forge strong partnerships with consumer and advocate groups. A second compilation of articles, beginning with "Who Are the Pioneers on the New Frontiers of Mental Health? Regional Responses to Changing Health Care Dynamics," features models of activists who are tenaciously meeting the demands of changing systems with innovation and vision. In our travels through uncharted territory, we may be guided by some of the latest technology, the Information Superhighway. Margaret Blodgett offers a preview of "The Internet and World Wide Web" and what it has to offer from the mental health vantage point.

The lead article, authored by Susan B. Fine, is "Surviving the Health Care Revolution: Rediscovering the Meaning of 'Good Work.'" It describes a somber landscape of dramatic changes in the social contract of health care with predictions of profound consequence for consumers, our patients, our practice and our professional self-image, as we struggle to reformulate our contributions in rapidly changing treatment contexts. It provides a much needed prescription for charting a path through the changing currents of health care reform, as we redefine ourselves from "victims to adventurers" (Noer, 1993) honing our survival skills.

CAN WE DELIVER WHAT WE PROMISE?

In an equally timely article, "Current and Future Education and Practice: Issues for Occupational Therapy Practitioners in Mental

Health Settings," the Mental Health Education Task Force, chaired by Deborah Walens, makes compelling recommendations that must be heeded if our specialty is to survive in the next century. This group forecasts that the clock is ticking and we are running out of time. All areas of occupational therapy practice are confronted with the crisis of packaging occupational therapy to meet the demands of the marketplace for economy, accountability and effectiveness. In mental health, the need for measurable, functionally-oriented treatment, documentation and outcomes that deliver what they promise is critical. Especially urgent, from my perspective, is the emphasis this report places on leadership and advocacy as primary survival skills. How well equipped are therapists trained at the baccalaureate level? Will the future ranks of occupational therapy students emerging from our educational programs be prepared for battle on the front lines of the health care revolution or be sidelined by passivity and conformity? In a prophetic publication, *Occupational Therapy; 2001* (1979), Yerxa spoke to the need for therapists to be not only nurturing caregivers, but also to be "self-directed, confident and highly visible . . . actively seek[ing] power . . . to create positive social change" (p. 28, 30). With our current models of education and practice, will we be ready to wield this power in the near future, so that we can still care for patients in 2001?

ONE LAST TIME NOW–WHAT IS OCCUPATIONAL THERAPY IN MENTAL HEALTH?

The Mental Health Education Task Force reports what most of us already knew; occupational therapists still do not agree upon a clear definition of our profession. If we do not define ourselves and what we do, then others will do it for us. Any ambiguity about our methods and goals will be used against us by those who feel we have no role to play in shaping the future of mental health. But it is not enough to let the world know who we are and what we do. We must also assert that our strategies are the ones which will achieve the best results for our consumers. We can be cost-efficient and still be humane. We can base our practice methods on scientific research; but foremost we must not lose sight of the dignity of every human being. We need to guard against approaches to medical care financing that "change people into body parts on a high-tech assembly line" (Moyers, 1993), and where disorders of the mind and spirit have no parity in this cost-cutting, bottom-line approach to health care funding.

GETTING BACK TO THE BASICS

What is the scope of basic training for the occupational therapy student of the twenty-first century? Will the therapist of the future be equipped to address body, mind and spirit as envisioned by the early pioneers of moral treatment and occupational therapy or will only the physical aspects of treatment prevail? As educational programs opt to make psychosocial fieldwork optional, what message will this convey? Students may not learn what they are not taught–no big surprise. If they are not tutored in the art of addressing the emotions of a person, their skills in handling the human response in any practice area will atrophy and be relegated to a footnote in some dusty annals of occupational therapy archives.

Left to their own resources, most therapists choose not to work with individuals who experience mental illness. Research in our own field confirms this (Lyons & Hayes, 1993). How do we address attitudes reflective of broader societal stereotypes. Is this even part of our educational and ethical mission? Exposure to mental health fieldwork can at least dispel some of the unfounded fears that occupational therapy students have related to working with the mentally ill, and at best it may lay a sound foundation for psychologically grounding students for future practice in all specialty areas.

The last constituency represented on the new frontiers is the work force of the future, occupational therapy students. Three students offer their views on psychosocial fieldwork and its impact on their education. In a companion piece, I present an approach to help students navigate their own emotional terrain of concerns in mental health settings, through using a learning contract based on Goal Attainment Scaling (GAS) (Kiresuk & Sherman, 1968; Scott & Haggerty, 1984; Scott, 1994) supported by an interactive log format.

Developing sensitivity to handling basic emotional states–fear, depression, anger, confusion, despair, denial, frustration, mistrust, elation–should be part of the basic training. All educational and most clinical programs espouse the philosophy of treating the whole person. If this is not happening, then we are all deceiving ourselves and we certainly are not educating the whole student to be a holistic practitioner. What goes in is what comes out, if we are only going to require students to work with broken limbs, then broken spirits will not be mended. We will perpetuate a standard of practice that supports technical excellence in a vacuum of psychological ignorance. Something as esoteric as spirituality and cultural sensitivity are now protected by JCAHO regulations. What we need is a patient's Bill of Rights in occupational therapy that demands attention to the whole person–not just the injured limb, symptom, or diagnostic category. Mental health as a practice area is under siege, and so is the rest of occupational therapy practice. We must heed the warnings–practice or perish, promise and deliver, and pioneer the new frontiers.

TAKING CHARGE OF OUR PROFESSIONAL DESTINY

The time has come when occupational therapists must play a leadership role in something no less than the direction and character of society. Will the much heralded "bridge to the 21st century" be accessible to individuals who use wheelchairs, or will we be told that it's too expensive to provide equal opportunities to all Americans? Will there be people sleeping under the "bridge" at night in cardboard boxes? Will some of us be afraid to cross the bridge and need reassurance? As politicians revel in metaphors about the future, let us not forget that we the people must tell the politicians our goals and our suggestions for achieving these goals. As we explore new and better ways of giving consumers quality care at affordable prices, occupational therapists must be the scouts who forge ahead in order to find the best path. Without the light provided by compassion and common sense, the bridge will only lead to darkness.

Never has there been a greater need for therapists to demonstrate the pioneering spirit and assume leadership for our profession, for our clientele and for the new frontiers to come. We must be guided by our roots in promoting action. For occupational therapy our time has come–it is truly now or never.

ACKNOWLEDGMENTS

I would like to thank my husband, Richard, for his inspiration, support and assistance in preparing this volume and in writing this article. I am indebted to all the authors, who so generously shared their work in making this book possible and to Mary Donohue for suggesting the theme of new frontiers and helping to launch this publication. I would gratefully like to acknowledge Ms. Jean Williams-Franks for her careful preparation of the manuscript, Mitch Fox and Nuntanee Satiansukpong for editorial assistance, Joyce Sabari for thoughtful suggestions, and Diane Tewfik, of the Mental Health Special Interest Group of the New York Metropolitan District of New York State Occupational Therapy Association, and all the members of our network for their dedicated commitment to mental health practice. Jenifer Plummer-Barrett assisted with the last portion of the preparation for this volume. She is a much appreciated assistant to Marie-Louise Blount and Mary Donohue.

REFERENCES

Kiresuk, T. J., & Sherman, R. E. (1968). Goal attainment scaling: A general method for evaluating comprehensive mental health programs. *Community Mental Health Journal, 4*: 443-453.

Lyons, M., & Hayes, R. (1993). Student perceptions of persons with psychiatric and other disorders. *American Journal of Occupational Therapy, 47*(6), 143-148.

Scott, A. (1994, July). *Achieving goals in therapy and education.* Paper presented at the meeting of the Canadian-American Occupational Therapy Association Annual Conference, Boston, MA.

Scott, A. H. & Haggerty, E. (1984). Structuring goals via goal attainment scaling in occupational therapy groups in partial hospitalization settings. *Occupational Therapy in Mental Health, 4* (2): 39-58.

Moyers, B. (1993, February 22-24). *Healing and the Mind.* Videorecording: Public Broadcasting Service.

Noer, D. M. (1993). *Healing the wounds. Overcoming the trauma of layoffs and revitalizing downsized organizations.* San Francisco: Jossey Bass.

Yerxa, E. (1979). The philosophical base of occupational therapy. *Occupational Therapy; 2001.* Rockville, MD: American Occupational Therapy Association, 18-24.

Surviving the Health Care Revolution: Rediscovering the Meaning of "Good Work"

Susan B. Fine, MA, OTR, FAOTA

SUMMARY. The ongoing turmoil in the health care system exacts a significant toll on consumers, providers and society. New paradigms for service and employment relationships pose a threat to professional and personal security. Understanding the dynamic phenomena in the system, as well as our own responses to these changes, can assist practitioners in overcoming barriers that undermine our future. Managing our feelings, developing perspective on the issues, adjusting expectations, acquiring skills that transcend medical necessity, and promoting the social contract in health care are recommended strategies for dealing with the crisis in confidence affecting health care professionals. *[Article copies available for a fee from The Haworth Document Delivery Service: 1-800-342-9678. E-mail address: getinfo@ haworthpressinc.com]*

INTRODUCTION

The approaching twenty-first century will likely bring with it a longing for "new beginnings" and the fulfillment of hopes and dreams. Looking to the future through the clouded lense of the past

---

Susan B. Fine is Director, Therapeutic Activities and Psychiatric Rehabilitation Services, New York Hospital-Cornell Medical Center, Payne Whitney Clinic and Westchester Divisions, 525 East 68th Street, Box 140, New York, NY 10021.

[Haworth co-indexing entry note]: "Surviving the Health Care Revolution: Rediscovering the Meaning of 'Good Work.'" Fine, Susan B. Co-published simultaneously in *Occupational Therapy in Mental Health* (The Haworth Press, Inc.) Vol. 14, No. 1/2, 1998, pp. 7-18; and: *New Frontiers in Psychosocial Occupational Therapy* (ed: Anne Hiller Scott) The Haworth Press, Inc., 1998, pp. 7-18. Single or multiple copies of this article are available for a fee from The Haworth Document Delivery Service [1-800-342-9678, 9:00 a.m. - 5:00 p.m. (EST). E-mail address: getinfo@haworthpressinc.com].

decade, however, will be more a test of our resilience than the product of romantic optimism. In reality, with the ongoing changes and turmoil in the health care system the year 2000 looms as an unsettling source of professional and personal anxiety.

Health care in the '90s has been a humbling and often frightening experience for both providers and consumers. The tempo and substance of services have been dramatically altered by fiscal constraints, the proliferation of managed care companies, and the restructuring of health care institutions. While some changes have been for the better, others have seriously eroded the integrity and accessibility of services for some of our neediest consumers. Downsizing, rightsizing, hospital mergers and closures, capitation plans–a reduction in services and manpower, no matter what the jargon–also represent serious challenges to our professional values and security. The lack of reimbursement parity for mental illness, and decreased numbers of occupational therapists practicing in mental health, confound the dilemma for our consumers, as well as for those of us who have a sustained commitment to this population.

While the greatest threats are felt in our everyday professional and personal activities, the issues associated with this health care revolution transcend our job, our clinic, and our profession. They have serious implications for society as a whole. The nation's low sense of social well-being, influenced by substance abuse, violence, dysfunctional families, poverty and homelessness, is inextricably linked to ongoing problems in the health care system. Tempting as it is, we cannot divorce one from the other.

In the face of this situation, the promise of the next century remains elusive. What lies beyond midnight on December 31, 1999? Will health care and occupational therapy only be defined–and diminished–by the hard, sharp realities of the marketplace? Or, will our worst fears be tempered by the emergence of respect for the human condition and the resources that enable individuals to overcome illness and disability and assume meaningful roles in society? Can such seemingly diverse perspectives co-exist? Will we reach beyond our everyday concerns and professional biases to address these problems? Attending to both the personal and global requires perspective–perspective that can assist us in applying the principles and practices of occupational therapy while looking beyond our discipline-specific interests to serve the greater good.

In this article, the author hopes to promote that perspective by exploring some of the dynamic issues that confound our experience with the changing health care system. The author believes that a greater understanding of the phenomena will enhance our abilities to survive and even prosper.

THE CONTEXT:
IS THIS HEALTH CARE REFORM OR REVENGE?

All of us, irrespective of our practice specialty are enmeshed in a complex and dysfunctional system, attempting to adapt to short-term and often short-sighted fixes, while anxiously awaiting more substantive and friendly reform. Don't hold your breath! We are in for a long siege of change and challenge that will continue to jeopardize many of our most closely held assumptions and methods of practice.

In the move from fee-for-service to managed care, economic survival and profit have become the most powerful factors directing health care. Major service systems are now shaped by those who pay the bills, not by those who provide or need the service. Budgetary, rather than patient-centered priorities, are the greatest force in institutional management and clinical decision making. Foto reminds us that "yesterday's revenue centers are today's cost centers . . . the profits of managed care organizations and other employers decrease everytime OT services are provided" (Hettinger, 1996, p. 19). Less continues to be viewed as more. Shorter and shorter lengths of hospital stay propel us from bed to bed as we address an offending limb or behavioral symptom, but not the individual. Think about the frequency with which we now ask: "What's their reimbursement?" Rather than, "Who is this person and what's his situation?" "What does she need to rebuild her life?" Quality and consumer satisfaction are emerging in the lexicon of managed care, but providers are straining to give meaning to these words when manpower and programs have been drastically reduced.

While the abuses of a bottom-line mentality must be challenged, the need for containment is also clear. The high costs of health care have outstripped the nation's inflationary rates for years. The uncontrolled health care binge of the last three decades is a troubling product of provider self-interest and inadequate governmental planning. Efforts to improve health care and control costs have also produced unfortunate results. De-institutionalization, a badly needed social policy of the 1960s aimed at returning state hospital patients to society, failed to transfer essential resources to the community to ensure reintegration and survival. We continue to see its aftermath on the streets of our urban centers. Similarly, the founding fathers of Medicaid and Medicare failed to consider rates of inflation, the aging of America, and the risks inherent in allowing totally unregulated physician fees. We will bear the burden of their short-sightedness well into the next century if constructive action is not taken soon.

It does not require a PhD in economics or health care policy, or the power of public office, to recognize that a social institution as complex as health care requires thorough long-range planning and intelligent monitoring. It cannot be transformed with simple-minded solutions that speak more to immediate economic, political and social pressures than to the longer-term realities and residuals of human illness, disability and poverty. The American affinity for quick relief as the preferred mode for solving significant social problems does not bode well for the future.

The failure of the Clintons' ambitious health care reform initiatives was as much a reflection of this "Tagamet" mentality as it was the Administration's difficulty translating a complicated vision into digestible soundbytes. The real issue is not that the Clinton plan was not launched, for it was not the only game in town, but that no thoughtful, comprehensive plan emerged. While bits and pieces of reform have taken hold, no legitimate long-term solutions for this deeply rooted problem are evident. These issues will not disappear while our politicians argue the pros and cons of local vs. federal control. Sadly, the problems with health care are part of the fabric of American life. In spite of our status as the world's richest nation–one that spends far more of its income on health care than any other–people in many other countries live longer and get more care than we do. Thirty-nine million people lack coverage, and care–for all but the most privileged–is continuing to deteriorate. Consider the following:

- State budgets, with more control over health care funding than ever before, threaten to disenfranchise those who need services the most. Brutal cuts have been held in abeyance because of the November election. How will the dismal proposals of '96 get translated in '97 and later?
- Access will continue to be constrained by persistent emphasis on "medical necessity" rather than on prevention, continuity of care, and a real understanding of the risks involved in underestimating the tenacity of acute symptoms and ongoing residuals of a major mental illness.
- A narrow focus on biological aspects of illness and health ignores social and psychological factors that influence outcome and ultimate costs of managing mental illness.
- The continued absence of public policy supporting equal access to health care will intensify cultural, language and racial barriers and provoke more tensions among the social classes.

Under these conditions, illness will continue to go undetected and untreated, disabilities will be ignored, and the productivity and quality of life of a significant proportion of Americans will be even more seriously compromised than they are now.

Yet there are those who reassure us that everything will be OK. Remember the special-interest rhetoric of "Don't try to fix something that's not broken?" Tell that to people whose independence and quality of life are constrained by insurance that reimburses for wheelchairs, but not for braces that permit ambulation. Think about that when you see the way pain and isolation can turn aging into anguish because of ineligibility for home care. Consider those with the residual impairments of chronic mental illness whose lives are valued at fewer and fewer outpatient visits each year.

This is the context of today's health care environment: a work in progress, a marketplace described as "knowing the price of everything, but the value of nothing," a system more obsessed with the immediate growth of product lines than with the long term welfare of people. I don't know about you, but to me *this feels far more like revenge than reform*!

FINDING AN ANTIDOTE FOR OUR CRISIS
IN CONFIDENCE AND IDENTITY

The risks in this rapidly changing environment are not limited to our patients. We also find ourselves with little control over important aspects of our lives: our work and our own health care. The most stressful aspect of the situation is the challenge to personal assumptions about ourselves and the structure of the world in which we live and work. The health care revolution has not only opened our eyes to the inequities of the system for others, it has made us far more aware of how vulnerable we are to the "re-engineering" frenzy that produces lay-offs and the loss of a safety net we have taken for granted. Many of us have grown up in institutional cultures that have "taken care" of employees in return for good work and loyalty. In today's organizations, there is a new reality: hospitals and agencies will not ensure long term employment, or nurture our careers and sense of self-worth as they have in the past. Our understanding of, and responsiveness to, this change in expectations is critical to our survival and ultimate sense of security.

However, even the "survivors" of restructured organizations suffer greatly. Noer's *Healing the Wounds* (1993) addresses the emotional and functional residuals of those who are left behind. "It begins with a deep sense of violation . . . [and] often ends with angry . . . and depressed employees consumed with their attempt to hold on to jobs that become devoid of joy, spontaneity and personal relevancy . . . with the organization attempting to thrive in a competitive environment with a risk-averse, depressed work force" (p. 3). When left unattended–as they often are–these feelings and behaviors can be damaging to both the individual and the organization. They fester and invariably undermine productivity, the quality of our efforts, and even our health.

Discussions with colleagues from all disciplines affirm this phenomena. The mushrooming of responsibilities with the inevitable challenge to one's sense of competency when the volume and tempo of critical problem-solving and decision-making defy the speed of lightening and our definitions of "good work" takes a great toll. Reductions in autonomy and influence are also commonplace as discipline-specific departments succumb to decentralized functional programs. The search for meaningful ways to use one's expertise and skills, and exert influence on the system, test the hardiest amongst us. They describe sleepless nights and despairing days, as they wait for the next round of lay-offs to occur. If there is energy to spare–they struggle to reinvent themselves, hoping to fit in somewhere. This cannot be viewed as a transitory blip on the screen of our careers. These upheavals and stressors will be ongoing; it is their unrelenting nature that makes them so difficult to deal with. Nonetheless, dealing with them must be a high priority for practitioners at all levels.

How are *you* dealing with them? Do you believe yourself to simply be a witness to this process? Are you monitoring what is going on, anticipating its impact on you and your setting? Are you prepared to manage the turmoil? Or are you struggling with fear, frustration, distrust, anger, sadness and guilt? Moving beyond these feelings, and the shock of these changes, is of utmost importance. Too many feel stuck and deeply vulnerable, a state that is neither healthy nor productive if sustained for too long. We increase our vulnerability and stress if we fail to mobilize the same healthy coping capacities we try to cultivate in our patients. We must actively appraise our situation to determine how much threat and how much promise it represents. We must gather information, identify alternate rewards and opportunities that capitalize on our knowledge and skills. And, we must manage our emotions by using the healthiest mechanisms available to us (e.g., humor, altruism), developing sources of social support with colleagues, and seeking guidance from experts when indicated (i.e., organizational consultants, career counselors, head hunters or psychotherapists). Ultimately, we must make hard decisions and take thoughtful action for ourselves, our colleagues, and those who need our expertise.

What keeps us from doing this with greater vigor? After all, as a group we are good task-centered problem-solvers. We know the process well, we just seem to be more comfortable putting it to work in protected traditional settings. We need to liberate ourselves from the acute care setting. While once the centerpiece of the system, it is rapidly moving to the margins. To survive and thrive in today's system, we need to open our eyes, look beyond the familiar, think bigger and differently, and take risks!

The personal and systemic barriers that keep us from applying our knowledge and clinical models to new environments, including social, political and organizational settings, must be overcome. To surmount them, we must begin by acknowledging the emotional stress we are experiencing. Although an obvious strategy given our area of specialization, it is difficult to own up to these feelings, particularly if you are in a leadership position. Nonetheless, we must find or create opportunities to share these feelings and concerns with colleagues so we can appropriately "grieve" the losses of people, roles and processes-*and move on.*

We also need to *free ourselves from old organizational dependencies and recapture a sense of control and self-esteem* by developing an entrepreneurial perspective, by acquiring skills that have currency in a marketplace not limited by medical necessity, by building a greater tolerance for discipline-neutral work without fear of losing our "uniqueness" or identity, and by *determining what "good work" means to us.*

Good work, a manifestation of our personal knowledge and skills, is done "to accomplish a task, not please the boss or impress the system" (Noer, 1993, p. 139). This new psychology of employment, borne from the dramatic shift in the covenant between employee and employer, actually represents a healthier adult adaptation to work. We might well begin to operationalize it by translating our particular knowledge and skills into methods that help our colleagues and workers in other industries make constructive transitions (Bridges, 1980), create visions for the future, and learn how to live organizational lives as adventurers and not victims (Noer, 1993).

Leaders in today's health care settings have been characterized as needing to be "meaning makers" (Drath & Palus, 1993, p. 190), they structure a confusing and ambiguous environment toward some unifying purpose. This embraces extraordinarily valuable and marketable skills that can emerge from the rank and file, as well as from designated leadership. If someone doesn't make the effort to give meaning to these upheavals and paradigm shifts, the emotional debris associated with them will become dead weights, holding back individual initiative and organizational innovation.

TAKING RESPONSIBILITY IN A SYSTEM
THAT HAS GONE AMOK

We are all losers in a battle for change and equity that pits large "corporate" entities (managed care companies, expanding health networks, Federal and State reimbursement systems) against the American people. Whatever else one might say about the current status of health care reform, there must be a continued effort to make purposeful changes that transcend special interests. Not only because the health care system *is* broken, but also because the problem reaches far beyond the delivery of treatment and rehabilitation services. It speaks to our willingness to acknowledge the human condition and take responsibility–in small and large ways–for a social institution that certainly seems to have gone amok.

While we bemoan the singular bottom-line focus and lack of attention to the quality of services, too few of us think about the larger questions affecting quality. Here too we are confronted by questions of "meaning and purpose." Giving meaning and purpose to our work with others is not merely a philosophical exercise. It is an essential aspect of building a more responsive and stable system for all of us. The threat to our purpose–a corrosive concern that we are not important enough to our patients and the system–is what makes the changing marketplace so painful and demoralizing to practitioners of all persuasions.

The pursuit of meaning and purpose, an innate and distinctive attribute of the human mind, is a powerful tool of the adaptive process. We seek meaning to create personal order. We try to understand events and situations in order to respond appropriately, direct our energies, solve problems, retain our sense of personal identity and integrity, and find comfort and satisfaction in our chosen activities. This process is no less important in developing a rational plan for a system that is tied to the most challenging of personal life experiences: illness and disability.

A critical part of the foundation of health care that has been chipped away is *the social contract*: our sense of responsibility for the human as well as the biological parts of illness and health; our commitment to what health care should be about, what caregivers should provide, and what consumers should commit to in their efforts to overcome disability and sustain health.

The absence of such a contract is evident in the consumer's everyday encounters with us and the system. Unfortunately, too many of us are defining rehabilitation–with all its individual promise and despair–by the clock and pocketbook, but not by the person. We are losing those powerful connections between patient and therapist that can transform traumas into triumphs–the kind of contract that cannot be clocked or bankrolled.

Fiscal constraints are not the only reasons we break our social contract. Humanistic approaches fall victim to shifts in scientific paradigms and political, religious and social attitudes. There is a troublesome parallel between the conditions that led to the demise of the 19th century Moral Treatment Era (an important antecedent of occupational therapy) and those influencing health care today. Today's emphasis on the biological determinants of mental illness with pressures to reimburse for medical necessity alone, battles over limited resources, and conflicts in accommodating to the increased cultural diversity of our country and our consumers are echoes of the past.

This health care crisis is in part a reflection of the larger crisis of class stratification and indifference in our society. Many Americans are driven principally by a personal interest in surviving–growing defensively indifferent to increasing problems of poverty, unemployment, violent crime and disrupted family lives that are major risk factors in sustaining health and adaptive function. We are so inundated by human tragedy and disregard for life that we sometimes fail to even notice the social toxicity in our own clinics.

Issues relating to meaning and purpose are at a critical crossroads–stretched between the same two competing belief systems that characterize the sides taken in the health reform debate: struggles between individualism and the greater good. Both can and must be nurtured and protected from the extremes of health care and political ideologies if we are to ever salvage the "American genius for consensus, for getting along by making up practical compromises to meet real social needs" (Hughes, 1993, p. 13-14). Let's hope that genius is merely dormant and not moribund. How far we are willing to go to revive it remains to be seen. There is an "underground" movement in health care, cutting across the often impenetrable boundaries between policy-makers, ethicists, providers and consumers (Lerner, 1993; McNerney, 1993; Osborne & Gaebler, 1990) that is attempting to gain a foothold in the marketplace. It speaks to the inner experience of the consumer; it asks about the meaning of our interventions with them and the way in which we use ourselves to influence outcomes. Service isn't simply giving someone something that they need in "a New York minute"; it is doing it in a way that empowers, gives dignity, and conveys a sense of caring and concern. Our encounters with our patients must reach beyond the behaviorally defined measures of function. "It is the face-to-face encounter, not the checklist or survey, this is needed" (Zoloth-Dorfman, 1993, p. 23). They also remind us that we share more with our patients than we care to admit. What we choose or promote for them, how well we listen and hear, how skillfully we advocate-must also be what we want for ourselves. "They" and "us" turn out to be "we" when it comes to coping with illness and changing the health care system (Fine, 1994; Fine, 1996).

All of this involves an expectation of a moral/ethical baseline that is not well represented in today's high-tech/high finance system. The pursuit of meaning and purpose is not easy. We have a great deal to lose, however, if the system continues unabashedly on one track. A morally bankrupt health care system will have little to offer occupational therapy and its consumers. On the other hand, responsive reform may bring the kind of changes we want-if we actively help mold its values, mission and priorities. The "underground" movement for meaning and purpose is a quiet and gentle one that needs our vision and the voices of similarly minded colleagues and consumers to give it the exposure and clout it deserves and needs.

Our vision, nurtured and revisited frequently since the first decade of this century, has always centered on the relationships between human activity and the meaning and purpose such activity provides for the individual. The same beliefs that have defined our work with individuals struggling with illness and disability, can define our relationship to the larger health care system and our communities-particularly as the boundaries of health care extend away from acute care centers to encompass prevention and health maintenance. While we continue to risk being all things to all people, our broad interactive biopsychosocial view of occupations and role performance can help prepare us to deal with the increasingly complex health care matrix.

CONCLUSION

We are poised between uncertainties: straddling the reality of a rapidly changing health care system and the questionable promise of a new century. This difficult situation requires major shifts in our assumptions about our work and our relationship to the system. Meeting the challenges of the year 2000 means plumbing the depths of our understanding of ourselves and the powerful dynamics at work in this process of change. While reordering our expectations, we must develop personal and practice skills that help us manage ongoing challenges and strengthen our confidence and independence in ways that are transferrable to diverse settings and roles.

We must use our adaptive capacities and talents to influence the evolving health care system in ways that reflect concern for the human condition as well as the bottom-line. By promoting and integrating the richness of our professional values and knowledge, we can bring substance to the system's preliminary efforts to redefine the meaning of "good work."

REFERENCES

Bridges, W. (1988). *Surviving corporate transitions: Rational management in a world of mergers, layoffs, start-ups, takeovers, divestitures, deregulations, and new technologies.* New York: Doubleday.

Drath, W. H., & Palus, C. J. (1993). *Leadership and meaning making in a community of practice.* Greensboro, N.C.: The Center for Creative Leadership, 1993.

Fine, S. B. (1994). *Finding meaning and purpose in reform: A challenge to our vision, knowledge and initiative.* Keynote address: Occupational Therapy Association of California Conference, Los Angeles.

Fine, S. B. (1996). The future of mental health practice. In M. Brinson & K. Kannenberg (Eds.) *Mental health service delivery guidelines.* Bethesda, MD: American Occupational Therapy Association.

Hettinger, J. (1996, May 9). Navigating in new frontiers. *OT Week,* p. 19.

Hughes, R. (1993). *The Culture of Complaint.* NY: Warner.

Lerner, M. (1993). Memos to Clinton: How to regain your popularity. *Tikkun,* *8*(4), 11-19.

McNerney, W. J. (1993). *Health care reform will not be enough.* Health Care Visions, 1(11), 1.

Noer, D. M. (1993). *Healing the wounds: Overcoming the trauma of layoffs and revitalizing downsized organizations.* San Francisco: Jossey-Bass.

Osborne, D., & Gaebler, T. (1990). *Reinventing government.* New York: Plume.

Zoloth-Dorfman, L. (1993). First, make meaning: An ethics of encounter for health care reform. *Tikkun, 8*(4), 23-26, 89.

Who Are the Pioneers
on the New Frontiers of Mental Health?
Regional Responses
to Changing Health Care Dynamics

Anne Hiller Scott, PhD, OTR, FAOTA

"Think globally and act locally" is a phrase often heard in political circles. The articles that follow illustrate how contemporary pioneers are meeting this challenge. Across the country, at the state and local level, mental health practitioners are uniting to preserve, protect and regenerate the vision of occupational therapy dedicated to meeting the needs of the mentally ill. From the East to the West, pioneering endeavors are underway. The next four articles feature several states–Kentucky, Wisconsin, California, and New York–in recognition of their progressive efforts.

With shrinking lengths of stay, funding constraints and emphasis on community-based treatment, therapists are challenged to effectively redefine their services and provide cost-effective models. Rather than be engulfed in the tumultuous changes which for some in health care have presaged lost frontiers, these therapists have chosen the route of action and discovery. In this journey therapists

Anne Hiller Scott is Director, Division of Occupational Therapy, School of Health Professions, Long Island University-Brooklyn Campus, 1 University Plaza, Brooklyn, NY 11201.

[Haworth co-indexing entry note]: "Who Are the Pioneers on the New Frontiers of Mental Health? Regional Responses to Changing Health Care Dynamics." Scott, Anne Hiller. Co-published simultaneously in *Occupational Therapy in Mental Health* (The Haworth Press, Inc.) Vol. 14, No. 1/2, 1998, pp. 19-20; and: *New Frontiers in Psychosocial Occupational Therapy* (ed: Anne Hiller Scott) The Haworth Press, Inc., 1998, pp. 19-20. Single or multiple copies of this article are available for a fee from The Haworth Document Delivery Service [1-800-342-9678, 9:00 a.m. - 5:00 p.m. (EST). E-mail address: getinfo@haworthpressinc.com].

are forging new partnerships with consumers, other disciplines and advocacy groups.

In Kentucky, occupational therapists are working at the state level with consumers, managed care and health care providers to formulate outcome measures related to function, as well as symptoms and consumer satisfaction. From Wisconsin, shifts to more community-based services linked with changes in patient demographics and acuity has promoted innovative programming in more client-centered models with occupational therapists assuming consultative and case management roles.

In California, the Psych Action Coalition has resolved in its mission statement to "revitalize the practice of psychiatric OT through education, information and advocacy for consumers, health care providers and the community." In New York City, the Mental Health Task Force has been forging alliances with consumers, monitoring legislative and regulatory efforts and is exploring one of the last frontiers of psychiatry–psychiatric home care.

By their example, therapists from these areas offer a broad range of venues for dealing with change from a proactive stance. As pioneers on the frontiers of mental health in our communities, we all have the potential to find new pathways for occupational therapy by thinking globally and acting locally!

Contributing to System Change in Kentucky: Occupational Therapy in an Evolving Program of Medicaid Managed Behavioral Healthcare

Lisette N. Kautzmann, EdD, OTR/L, FAOTA

SUMMARY. Currently a change that requires monitoring and action is the state public payers' movement toward managed behavioral health care and the re-structuring of Medicaid to reflect this movement. In this article the response of one state, Kentucky, to managing Medicaid costs, quality and access is reported. The author's participation in a multi-disciplinary effort to identify outcomes and outcome measures for the state's managed behavioral healthcare system is described. The proposed Medicaid waiver for mental health and substance abuse and the resulting implications for occupational therapy are discussed. *[Article copies available for a fee from The Haworth Document Delivery Service: 1-800-342-9678. E-mail address: getinfo@haworth pressinc.com]*

Over two decades, authors have called attention to the diminishing number of occupational therapists in mental health settings (Ethridge, 1976; American Occupational Therapy Association (AOTA), 1984;

Lisette N. Kautzmann is Professor, Department of Occupational Therapy, Dizney 103, Eastern Kentucky University, Richmond, KY 40475.

[Haworth co-indexing entry note]: "Contributing to System Change in Kentucky: Occupational Therapy in an Evolving Program of Medicaid Managed Behavioral Healthcare." Kautzmann, Lisette N. Co-published simultaneously in *Occupational Therapy in Mental Health* (The Haworth Press, Inc.) Vol. 14, No. 1/2, 1998, pp. 21-28; and: *New Frontiers in Psychosocial Occupational Therapy* (ed: Anne Hiller Scott) The Haworth Press, Inc., 1998, pp. 21-28. Single or multiple copies of this article are available for a fee from The Haworth Document Delivery Service [1-800-342-9678, 9:00 a.m. - 5:00 p.m. (EST). E-mail address: getinfo@haworthpressinc.com].

1991, 1995; Wittman, Swinehart, Cahill, & St. Michel, 1989; Paul, 1996, Scott 1990). Various reasons have been given for this phenomena: changes in practice preference, shrinking in-patient caseloads, lack of concreteness associated with mental health occupational therapy practice, and intense recruiting and high salaries offered in rehabilitation and long term care facilities. Until recently, efforts at the national level to curb the movement away from mental health practice have been sporadic. However, recent work undertaken by the American Occupational Therapy Association (AOTA) and the Steering Committee of the Mental Health Special Interest Section (MHSIS), including workshops on documentation and consultation, the completion and publication of the MHSIS Education Task Force Report (AOTA, 1995), publication of the position paper on "The Psychosocial Core of Occupational Therapy" (Commission on Practice, 1995a) and the statement "Psychosocial Concerns within Occupational Therapy Practice" (Commission on Education, 1995b), development of practice guidelines for schizophrenia, and passage by the Representative Assembly of Resolution A, "Mental Health and Psychosocial Issues within Occupational Therapy" (Brown, 1996), have provided direction and hope for a revitalization of mental health practice.

While support for mental health practice at the national level is critical, there also is need for state and local involvement in influencing political, reimbursement, and hiring decisions affecting occupational therapy. State associations and individual therapists must be vigilant in monitoring the external environment for proposed changes that have the potential to affect mental health practice, and in taking action to influence the change. Since individual clinicians and their practice settings frequently are tenuously linked to decision-makers at higher levels, it is important for therapists to understand the system in which they work, as well as other external forces that have the potential to impact that system.

Currently a change that requires monitoring and action is the state public payers' movement toward managed behavioral healthcare and the re-structuring of Medicaid to reflect this movement. While at the national level health care reform has moved forward slowly, states have recognized and responded to the need to take action quickly to stem the increasing cost of Medicaid. Medicaid spending has doubled since 1987 (VanLeit, 1996) and now constitutes a significant portion of states' budgets. As a result, a number of states are moving to Medicaid managed care. In order to move to a system of managed care for Medicaid recipients, states must apply to the Health Care Financing Administration for waivers from Medicaid regulations. The focus of this article will be on the response of one state, Kentucky, to the crisis in Medicaid, including the proposed Medicaid waiver for mental health and substance abuse and the resulting implications for occupational therapy.

THE KENTUCKY PLAN

In Kentucky, legislation passed in 1994 mandated establishment of a management and oversight system to improve the state's Medicaid program. When this legislation was passed, Kentucky was spending 51% of its Medicaid mental health dollars on child and adult inpatient or residential services (Division of Mental Health, 1995a). This figure was seen as disproportionate to the actual need for this type of restrictive care. Provided services were driven by a fee for service mechanism rather than by individual needs. Additionally, services to recipients were "weighted heavily toward inpatient care and outpatient services with gaps in intermediate levels of care and crisis stabilization services" (Division of Mental Health, 1995a, p. 1).

The waiver submitted to HCFA by the Kentucky Cabinet for Health Services proposes a "carve out" of mental health services with administration and oversight of these services delegated to the SMHA. In addition to cost containment through capitated payment, payers, who reimburse service providers, are required to monitor process and outcome measures related to consumer access to quality, effective services (Littrell, 1997). The objective of the proposed management system is to provide a seamless system of inpatient and outpatient mental health and substance abuse service delivery.

To facilitate development of process and outcome measures, a Managed Mental Health Outcomes Committee was appointed. Since SMHA strongly believed that identification of key outcomes should include input from all stakeholders, a variety of groups, agencies and organizations representing consumers and their families, providers, legislators, university faculty and SMHA staff were invited to participate. To expedite the selection of measures for the identified outcomes, committee members were assigned to sub-groups representing each of the four categories of service consumers: adults with severe mental illness; adults with general mental health problems; children and adolescents; and substance abusing adults. Each committee then discussed which of the identified outcomes were the most critical for the identified population. Following the discussion, a number of outcome measurement instruments were reviewed.

Results of the sub-groups' deliberations indicated consensus that no one instrument would address all required outcomes. Therefore multiple instruments were recommended. At that time (April, 1996) the Mental Health Statistics Improvement Program (MHSIP) Task Force released the final draft of it's *Consumer-Oriented Mental Health Report-Card*. Since there were multiple similarities between the Committee recommendations and the MHSIP Report Card, an administrative decision was made to adopt the MHSIP measures in areas that were significantly similar. The identified domains of concern were: access; quality; effectiveness; prevention; and cost. Measures to assess outcomes were grouped broadly into two categories: satisfaction surveys and clinical assessment instruments.

GETTING A VOICE IN MANAGED BEHAVIORAL HEALTHCARE

Kentucky is a state that has a long history of un-met personnel needs. Although there has been a recent influx of new therapists, the positions that they have been recruited for have been primarily in the areas of rehabilitation and long term care. In terms of mental health, there have been well-established occupational therapy departments in the state hospital system since the 1920's. However, when the move toward de-institutionalization occurred, therapists did not follow their patients into the community. Community-based services to Medicaid recipients are provided through programs directed by the 14 regional mental health/mental retardation boards. Occupational therapists unfortunately have never been employed in these community-based programs. Additionally, there has been little interaction between the state hospitals and the regional community-based programs. Therefore, when the Division of Mental Health Services (DMHS) of the Kentucky Department of Mental Health and Mental Retardation Services announced the proposed Medicaid waiver for services to adults with serious mental illness, substance abusing adults, persons with intermittent mental illness, and children and adolescents, this was seen as an opportunity to work towards expanding opportunities for provision of occupational therapy services to these consumers.

However, since occupational therapy is not viewed by the state mental health system as a profession that typically provides treatment to persons who are mentally ill or substance abusers, occupational therapists were not included in the initial invitation to participate in the outcomes development. This was remedied when the author requested and received an appointment to the Committee, serving on both the Technical Advisory Group and the Adults with Severe Mental Illness Subcommittee. A concurrent priority was to assure that occupational therapy services would be paid for under the new managed care plan. The language of the proposed waiver expands the state's statutory definition of "qualified mental health professional" to include licensed and certified behavioral health professionals (DMHS, 1995b). Verification, through the State Practice Act, that occupational therapists met the expanded definition was accomplished through personal and written communication with SMHA.

DISCUSSION

Moving to an outcome-based, capitated managed behavioral healthcare system will drastically affect all areas of service. While mandated program components such as access to case management services, availability of in-patient and community-based care, family education, etc., will still be available to consumers, the emphasis will be on selecting the appropriate mix of program components to meet each consumer's needs (DMHS, 1995b). This approach opens the door for new, innovative methods of service delivery. Programs for all of the targeted groups rely heavily on counseling and symptom management, with minimal emphasis on functional performance. In managed behavioral healthcare, functional performance in all three occupational therapy domains, self-care, work, and leisure will be scrutinized. Through participating in the discussions, it became apparent that occupational therapists were the professionals that understood function and implications of impaired function most clearly. In addition, consumers and family are supportive of outcome measures related to function. Lastly, function was the major issue at the most recent consumer conference in the state. Therefore, there is reason for optimism regarding future opportunities to expand provision of occupational therapy services to Medicaid recipients in both public and private programs. Consumers want to become more functional and traditional service providers are not as skillful in these areas as occupational therapists; their strengths are in symptom management and counseling.

Service delivery that addresses outcomes predictably will be different than traditional practice. In Kentucky, the proposed decreases in in-patient length of stay will result in fewer opportunities for therapists in these settings. However, since most of the treatment will occur in the community, there will be demands for services that result in achievement of outcomes related to functional performance. In a controlled study at Fort Bragg, North Carolina it was found that even when all of the access, cost and quality measures of a managed behavioral healthcare program were in place, the outcomes did not improve because *the service delivery programs did not change* [italics added] (Bickman, 1996). Occupational therapists can provide these services directly, particularly in collaboration with a Certified Occupational Therapy Assistant (COTA), or as a consultant to multiple programs.

CONCLUSION

The language of the proposed waiver, which describes a health care system that is flexible, comprehensive, and cost effective in a continuum of settings, (VanLeit, 1996) clearly speaks to an intent of implementing a third generation approach to managed care. As a result, there is a window of opportunity for occupational therapists to expand mental health practice. Currently, there are gaping holes in the services available to help people become more functional.

Occupational therapists have the skills to bridge those gaps by focusing on functional performance–the expansion of valued roles in self-care, work, and play/leisure.

In marketing our services it is important to focus on the achievement of functional outcomes rather than duplicating what others may be doing, even if it is within our practice domain. By taking this approach we will be viewed as assets to new and existing programs, rather than threats. This is a time for building alliances and networking with other professionals and consumer organizations.

ACKNOWLEDGMENTS

The author would like to acknowledge the following people for their assistance and support: Robert Littrell, PharmD, Chair and Richard Heine, PhD, Co-Chair, Managed Care Outcomes Committee; members of the sub-committee on Adults with Severe Mental Illness; Marian Kavanagh Scheinholtz, MS, OTR, AOTA, Mental Health Program Manager; and Joy Anderson, MA, OTR/L, FAOTA, Professor, Department of Occupational Therapy, Eastern Kentucky University.

REFERENCES

American Occupational Therapy Association (1984). *1982 Member data survey–Final report.* Rockville, MD: Author.

American Occupational Therapy Association (1991). *1990 Member data survey.* Rockville, MD: Author.

American Occupational Therapy Association (March, 1995). *Mental health special interest section education task force report.* Bethesda, MD: Author.

Bickman, L. (1996). A continuum of care: More is not always better. *American Psychologist, 51* 689-701.

Brown, E. J. (1996, May 6). RA passes resolution A: Psych to get new emphasis in classroom and clinic. *ADVANCE for Occupational Therapists,* p. 3.

Commission on Practice (1995a). [Position paper] The psychosocial core of occupational therapy. *American Journal of Occupational Therapy, 49,* 1021-1022.

Commission on Practice (1995b). [Statement] Psychosocial concerns within occupational therapy practice. *American Journal of Occupational Therapy, 49,* 1011-1013.

Division of Mental Health Services. (1995a, September 15). *Executive summary, Kentucky ACCESS: Assuring continuity of care through an effective mental health and substance abuse service system* [Draft]. Frankfort, KY: Author.

Division of Mental Health Services. (1995b, September 15). *Kentucky ACCESS:*

Assuring continuity of care through an effective mental health and substance abuse service system [Draft]. Frankfort, KY: Author.

Ethridge, D. A. (1976). The management view of the future of occupational therapy in mental health. *American Journal of Occupational Therapy, 30*, 623-628.

Littrell, R. (1997, March 28). *Working for results*. Mental Health Managed Care Outcomes Committee Report. Frankfort, KY: Kentucky Department of Mental Health and Mental Retardation Services.

Paul, S. (1996). [The issue is] Mental health: An endangered occupational therapy specialty? *American Journal of Occupational Therapy, 50*, 65-68.

Scott, A. H. (1990). A review, reflections and recommendations: Specialty preference of mental health in occupational therapy. *Occupational Therapy in Mental Health, 10* (1), 1-20.

VanLeit, B. (1996). Managed mental health care: Reflections in a time of turmoil. *American Journal of Occupational Therapy, 50*, 428-434.

Wittman, P. P., Swinehart, S., Cahill, R., & St. Michel, G. (1989). Variables affecting specialty choice in occupational therapy. *American Journal of Occupational Therapy, 43*, 602-606.

Responsive Changes
in Mental Health Practice in Wisconsin

Linda Samuel, MS, OTR

SUMMARY. Delivery of mental health care is changing dramatically at the state and county levels in Wisconsin. These new trends are affecting psychiatric institutions and rehabilitation personnel in reference to staffing patterns, the roles of occupational therapists, certified occupational therapy assistants, patient population and level of acute care and the type and site of intervention. Therapists are moving to more community-based and innovative programming and are leading state and local advocacy initiatives.

Many occupational therapists in Wisconsin have become pioneers pursuing nontraditional occupational therapy roles in response to changes in philosophy, funding, population demographics and evolving needs. *[Article copies available for a fee from The Haworth Document Delivery Service: 1-800-342-9678. E-mail address: getinfo@haworthpressinc.com]*

CHANGES IN THE MISSION
AND SERVICES OF THE STATE

The delivery of mental health care is being changed at the state level in Wisconsin. The Mental Health Bureau of Health and Family Services (MHBHFS) is redesigning its long term care system and mental health delivery to ensure that "persons in need of tax sup-

---

Linda Samuel is Assistant Professor, Concordia University, 12800 North Lake Shore Drive, Mequon, WI 53097.

[Haworth co-indexing entry note]: "Responsive Changes in Mental Health Practice in Wisconsin." Samuel, Linda. Co-published simultaneously in *Occupational Therapy in Mental Health* (The Haworth Press, Inc.) Vol. 14, No. 1/2, 1998, pp. 29-34; and: *New Frontiers in Psychosocial Occupational Therapy* (ed: Anne Hiller Scott) The Haworth Press, Inc., 1998, pp. 29-34. Single or multiple copies of this article are available for a fee from The Haworth Document Delivery Service [1-800-342-9678, 9:00 a.m. - 5:00 p.m. (EST). E-mail address: getinfo@haworthpressinc.com].

ported mental health services are provided with access to appropriate, high quality and cost-effective services that promote health and wellness, improvement and recovery, and quality of life" (Executive Order No. 282, 1996, p. 1). A Governor's Blue Ribbon Commission in Mental Health Care is developing mission and vision statements and will work in a parallel fashion with MHBHFS.

Winnebago Mental Health Institute (WMHI) is a facility that provides treatment for persons with mental illness located in northern Wisconsin, with an average daily census of 240. Wayne Winistorfer (personal communication, August, 1996), the clinical director of Rehabilitative Services at Winnebago, identifies three major trends at this facility. First, admissions of forensic consumers has increased with half currently entering Winnebago through the legal system, as growing numbers of the chronic mentally ill are being charged with crimes and deemed incompetent to stand trial. They require treatment until evaluated as competent or require placement until they can be safely returned to the legal system or the community. In addition, some forensic consumers arrive from other counties of the state, which lack the resources to manage the behavioral treatment requirements of the forensic population. A second trend is an increasing population of dually diagnosed consumers including those with mental illness with drug/alcohol abuse or developmental disabilities and mental illness and a physical illness (HIV or tuberculosis). Finally, the consumers at WMHI are admitted with more acute symptoms and severe loss of function.

These changes in consumer populations and levels of acute symptoms have altered rehabilitation staffing patterns. Over the past year the rehabilitation staff has increased by one third to 55 persons composed of equal numbers of registered occupational therapists, certified occupational therapy assistants (COTAs) and recreational therapists. Occupational therapists administer standardized evaluations: the Allen Cognitive Level (ACL) (Allen, Earhart, & Blue, 1992), the Allen Diagnostic Module (ADM) (Earhart, Allen & Blue, 1993), and the Milwaukee Evaluation of Daily Living Skills (MEDLS) (Leonardelli, 1988). A variety of other assessments are also used to quickly and objectively measure functional deficits. The occupational therapists at WMHI also provide diverse types of group treatment. Vocational programs are instituted, ranging from sheltered work to community integration, and these are often led by COTAs. Therapists recognize the need to communicate effectively with community institutions to promote community integration since many consumers are working in the community at supported settings.

The county of Milwaukee is considered demographically unique within Wisconsin. Its population is largely over the age of 18 with approximately 24% of the population over the age of 60. It is culturally diverse: 75% of the population is white, 20% of the population is African-American, 2% is Asian and Pacific Islander, 1% is Native American and 2% other races. In the city of Milwaukee, the nation's 17th largest city, only 63% of the population is Caucasian (Executive Summary, DHS, 1992). Milwaukee County is currently at a crossroads in determining the future of the delivery of mental health services. The mental health treatment needs of this diverse county are provided at Milwaukee County Mental Health Complex (MCMHC).

At MCMHC, located in the southeast part of the state, the number of inpatient beds and staff are decreasing as a result of the reorganization of the Department of Human Services. In 1991, as a second phase of this reorganization, a five year Master Plan was developed for the public sector mental health services for adults residing in Milwaukee County, with a vision of incorporating people with mental illness as contributing members of the community. The service system consists of an array of community resources to decrease the need for inpatient services. These community services include: risk reduction programs (public mental health referral/education), wellness/rehabilitative services (day hospital, outpatient clinics, drop-in centers, etc.), pre-crisis services (respite, homeless programs, etc.), crisis response (mobile crisis unit, psychiatric crisis service hotline, etc.), and inpatient services. The goal is to decrease the number of consumers receiving inpatient services. In 1992, the total bed capacity was 575 at MCMHC and the goal is to decrease that number to 245 by 1997.

As a result of the Master Plan, MCMHC is already undergoing a downsizing of staff. In 1989, there were 150 rehabilitation staff employed at MCMHC. Of these, 80 were registered occupational therapists and 50 were COTAs. Today the number of rehabilitation staff has been cut by approximately half, with a total of 40 occupational therapists and 18 COTAs being employed. One quarter of the current staff is now working in the community.

NONTRADITIONAL POSITIONS
FOR OCCUPATIONAL THERAPISTS

To adapt to the changing health care arena in psychiatry, many occupational therapists in Wisconsin are developing nontraditional positions. To qualify as a case manager, Wisconsin requires a bachelor's degree and two years of experience. Kathi Zarwell, OTR, (personal communication, August, 1996), a former employee of MCMHC, applied for a case management position that was formerly held by a registered nurse. As a case manager for mentally ill consumers in Waukesha County for the past 8 years, she monitors the fiscal affairs of the consumers and must be aware of community resources, as well as medication issues. In addition, she advocates for the consumers to obtain needed treatment and presents evaluations in court for commitment/guardian hearings.

John Chianelli, OTR (personal communication, August, 1996), works in the Service Access to Independent Living (SAIL) Program at MCMHC, with a primary role of coordination of services. He has employed his occupational therapy skills in completing functional assessments, communicating with varied disciplines assisting with placement and finalizing contracts with case management agencies.

Mary Jo Kostan, OTR (personal communication, August, 1996), was working for Milwaukee County, at the Child and Adolescent Treatment Center (CATC) when the program received a federal seed grant to begin an integrated service project providing in-home treatment for families with children who have severe emotional problems. The goal of this project was to decrease hospitalization stays and placement outside of the home using a multidisciplinary approach. Subsequently, CATC was awarded a 15 million dollar grant for a five year project. Ms. Kostan assumed the role of program coordinator for therapeutic case management and most recently has been promoted to assistant project director. As an occupational therapist, Ms. Kostan found that she has had to display confidence in herself in order to supervise other disciplines, be comfortable with a multidisciplinary approach and oversee agencies that contract with children and families.

In September of 1996, two occupational therapists, Janet Arnold and Kathy Miller (personal communication, August, 1996) from Milwaukee County became coordinators at the Grand Avenue Club in downtown Milwaukee. These positions are funded by Milwaukee County. The Grand Avenue Club follows the Fountain House Model and as members these occupational therapists will be involved in the creation of new vocational programs assisting club members with practical skills. As occupational therapists, they will need to adjust to a nonmedical model and use their occupational therapy skills in the role of members rather than therapists. This creates a challenge for them and both are excited about exploring this new realm of nontraditional practice.

MENTAL HEALTH TASK FORCE ADVOCACY

The Wisconsin Occupational Therapy Association (WOTA) has responded to changes in mental health services by providing increased education to its members and forming a Mental Health Task Force in 1990. The task force grew out of the need to have a voice within the legislature to insure the inclusion of occupational therapy. The task force provides a day long workshop on mental health issues every two years and is currently networking with mental health groups from other states. A brochure titled, *Occupational Therapy: Makes Good Sense for Case Management* was developed by the Mental Health Task Force to promote occupational therapists as case managers. WOTA has also sponsored workshops on mental health issues and included pertinent topics at the State WOTA Conference.

Mental health practice is changing in the state of Wisconsin. Occupational therapists are responding effectively by adjusting staffing patterns, adapting treatment for more acute populations and having the foresight to explore nontraditional avenues of occupational therapy.

REFERENCES

Allen, C., Earhart, C., & Blue, T. (1992). *Occupational therapy treatment goals for the physically and cognitively disabled.* Rockville, MD: American Occupational Therapy Association.

Earhart, C., Allen, C., & Blue, T. (1993). *Allen diagnostic module.* Colchester, CT: S&S Worldwide.

Executive Order 282, (1996). The State of Wisconsin.

Executive summary, master plan for the public sector adult mental health system in Milwaukee county. (1992). Department of Human Services, Wisconsin.

Leonardelli, C. (1988). *Milwaukee evaluation of daily living skills.* Thorofare, NJ: Slack.

Advocacy, Partnerships
and Client Centered Practice in California

Jane Dressler, MA, OTR
Anne MacRae, PhD, OTR

SUMMARY. This article highlights the many accomplishments of California based mental health occupational therapists in fostering liaisons in the community, collaborating with consumers and families and developing innovative programs. It also provides a rationale and theoretical construct for occupational therapists to provide quality interventions while both protecting and expanding their present practice through the use of client centered services. *[Article copies available for a fee from The Haworth Document Delivery Service: 1-800-342-9678. E-mail address: getinfo@haworthpressinc.com]*

Occupational therapists working in mental health settings in California's San Francisco Bay Area have a long history of activism. A group known informally as the "OT Psych Forum" began in the early 1980's for the purposes of continuing education, networking, and promotion of mental health practice. For years the group met monthly at local hospitals with good attendance. In 1995, taking the cue from a New York State occupational therapy mental

---

Jane Dressler is affiliated with San Francisco General Hospital, Department of Psychiatry and Occupational Therapy, 1001 Potero Avenue, San Francisco, CA 94110.

Anne MacRae is Associate Professor, San Jose State University, College of Applied Sciences and Arts, Department of Occupational Therapy, One Washington Square, San Jose, CA 95192-0059.

[Haworth co-indexing entry note]: "Advocacy, Partnerships and Client Centered Practice in California." Dressler, Jane, and Anne MacRae. Co-published simultaneously in *Occupational Therapy in Mental Health* (The Haworth Press, Inc.) Vol. 14, No. 1/2, 1998, pp. 35-43; and: *New Frontiers in Psychosocial Occupational Therapy* (ed: Anne Hiller Scott) The Haworth Press, Inc., 1998, pp. 35-43. Single or multiple copies of this article are available for a fee from The Haworth Document Delivery Service [1-800-342-9678, 9:00 a.m. - 5:00 p.m. (EST). E-mail address: getinfo@haworthpressinc.com].

health special interest group (Tewfik, 1995), and responding to issues related to managed care, health care reform, behavioral health care systems, the need to demonstrate functional outcomes, and the decreasing numbers of occupational therapists working in mental health settings, the informal OT Psych Forum decided to become more formal, more assertive and more action-oriented. This group is now known as the "Psychiatric Occupational Therapy Action Coalition" (POTAC) and has adopted the mission of "revitalizing the practice of psychiatric occupational therapy through education, information and advocacy for consumers, health care providers and the community."

The group is 120 members strong, headed by a steering committee of five occupational therapists, and is dedicated to printing a quarterly newsletter, planning and convening one to two full day symposiums and five two hour Friday afternoon educational forums a year, as well as coordinating the work of "action committees." These committees are involved with projects such as lobbying for mental health resources, research and publication, advocacy, program development, education, and publicity.

The work of this group is inspired by and based upon the principles of client centered mental health practice as articulated by the Canadian Association of Occupational Therapists (CAOT) and Law, Baptiste and Mills (1995). The CAOT publication, *Occupational Therapy Guidelines for Client Centered Mental Health Practice* (1993), discussed many important concepts that this article's authors have grouped into two key areas. The first area addresses empowering the client and the second addresses adapting and changing the environment. A third area not explicitly covered in the CAOT document but critical to the work of POTAC members is forming partnerships.

EMPOWERING THE CLIENT

In traditional medical and rehabilitation models, practitioners are seen as care givers, goals are set for clients and things are done for them. In a Client Centered Practice (CCP), a partnership is formed to help clients enhance functioning in self-care, productivity and leisure. Therapists work with clients to develop skills, habits and volition necessary to gain power to make decisions and to take action in their lives. Most importantly in a CCP, clients set their own goals. Clients are seen as active agents and participants in their treatment. They are considered experts regarding their needs and the primary decision makers (CAOT, 1993). Glenda Jeong, an occupational therapist and director of a community-based vocational service program, uses the metaphor of an airplane–she is the navigator–the clients are the pilots (Tapper, 1996). Jerry Veverka, president of the California Alliance for the Mentally Ill (CAMI) asks that all mental health practitioners begin with what people want for themselves (J. Vererka, 1996). Realistically, in current practice it is not unheard of, or even uncommon for treatment plans to be written without clients' input. In a CCP, this is no longer acceptable practice.

CCP does not negate the importance of professional expertise, but is guided by a commitment to listen and respond to each client. The clients' personal knowledge and experience of living with a mental illness enable them to explain their lives, goals and plans and allows them to seek personal meaning in their lives. Clients must be given the opportunity for making real choices and therapists must be sensitive to potential for dominating clients by virtue of professional position and knowledge (CAOT, 1993).

In mental health settings there is typically much discussion about client compliance with treatment regimes. If a person is not complying, one must ask if the client's goals are being addressed (Bowen, 1996). If client goals are vague or unrealistic, probing interview questions can be used to clarify and quantify goals. Therapists may feel uncomfortable with client choices, but must learn to strike a balance between explaining choices and assisting, influencing and protecting clients from making choices. The clients right to take risks must be respected (CAOT, 1993).

The Canadian Occupational Performance Measure (COPM) (Law, Baptiste, Carswell, McColl, Polatakjo, & Pollack, 1994) is an excellent client-centered assessment tool that identifies and evaluates problem areas in occupational performance and the client's satisfaction relative to these areas. The COPM consists of a semi-structured interview and rating scales to determine the client's self perception of occupational performance (Pollock, 1993). It can be used as an initial assessment, an outcome measure, an integral part of treatment, and as a tool to describe the domain of occupational therapy.

Occupational therapists in mental health often work with clients that have been rejected and dismissed and who have little hope, control, resources or social structures for making changes. The main focus of occupational therapy is to change the client's personal sense of unworthiness or helplessness to one of empowerment, control and fulfillment. Occupational therapists have traditionally done this by supporting clients in taking small practical steps as they engage in occupations and reflecting on the process through discussion of the experience. We must also strive to involve clients as much as possible in designing as well as participating in programs and in advocating for additional services. Needs assessments, program evaluation and client satisfaction surveys must be a routine part of practice. Current mental health practice is consumer oriented and there is a trend to include clients in the entire range of clinical, educational and research activities. Clark, Scott, and Krupa (1993) describe using this methodology in a study of client satisfaction. They concluded that "Involving clients in all aspects of planning, including clinical decision-making, programme development and evaluation, and research must become a priority in order that occupational therapy remain meaningful to clients, and their treatment" (p. 197).

ADAPTING AND CHANGING THE ENVIRONMENT

Occupational therapists using a CCP approach have two important roles in terms of adapting and changing environments. The first may be more familiar and focuses on the client's immediate environment. Occupational therapists are skilled in evaluating environments and either find the best match for a client or alter it to allow the person to function optimally. The uniqueness of an occupational therapy approach to environmental adaptation is rooted in occupational performance. Rather than simply attending to the physical environment, occupational therapists are aware of and address all of the occupational performance components–physical, psychological, sociocultural and spiritual–in an evaluation of the environment. Environmental adaptation obviously applies to the clinical setting but it also applies to the community. In mental health settings the occupational therapist typically develops or makes referrals to specialized living situations and vocational services that are structured for success. Educating family members and care givers in the amount and type of assistance a client may need is another familiar role and form of environmental adaptation. In order to accomplish community environmental adaptation, occupational therapists must be sensitive to the issues of the family. As stated by Peternelj-Taylor and Hartley (1993) "It is important for professionals working with the mentally ill to recognize the strength of families, and the tremendous burden that they cope with on a daily basis" (p. 27). Several members of POTAC have instituted specific groups for families within their clinical settings for the purposes of education and support.

The second way of adapting and changing the environment in a CCP focuses on the larger environment and asks therapists to pay attention to larger systems. This includes the role of the academic programs in preparing future occupational therapists. *The Client Centered Mental Health Practice* guidelines make a clear recommendation that public relation materials, fieldwork education and refresher education be specifically designed to attract individuals to occupational therapy mental health practice (CAOT, 1993). All San Francisco Bay Area occupational therapy schools are represented by instructors on the POTAC steering committee. The group has worked to expand mental health field work sites by placing students in non-traditional community based mental health settings and by training students in pairs and trios.

Occupational therapists also have a responsibility to ensure that clients have access to community, hospital and professional resources, and follow-up services in all programs. Our responsibility also includes advocating for and with clients to extend service mandates to fill gaps and ensure linkages between programs. Occupational therapists must also work to change social conditions like stigma and inequities, as well as environmental conditions that have detrimental effects on mental health (CAOT, 1993). These responsibilities led POTAC members to place special emphasis on the role of partnerships between organizations, disciplines, clients, family members, policy makers and legislators.

FORMING PARTNERSHIPS

Preserving and enhancing the profession's ability to provide quality psychiatric services is the preeminent concern of occupational therapists in mental health practice. One way to not only survive but flourish in these difficult times is to form partnerships with others who have a vested interest in supporting a quality mental health care system (Lang, Kannenberg, & Brinson, 1992). An often overlooked source of support for occupational therapy is the families of people with mental illness and clients themselves! But all too often people do not know about the role of OT, therefore they cannot possibly support it. Partnerships go both ways: Families of people with mental illness and clients with mental illness can be powerful spokespersons for the value of occupational therapy, but we as occupational therapists must be their visible and vocal advocates.

The Psychiatric Occupational Therapy Action Coalition (POTAC) of the San Francisco Bay area has made a tremendous effort in the area of linkage with families and clients. Members are active in the National Alliance for the Mentally Ill (NAMI), a family, client and professional organization dedicated to advocacy for the severely mentally ill, as well as board members of local AMI affiliates and presenters at the California Alliance for the Mentally Ill annual conference. POTAC members are involved with self-help groups such as the Depressive/Manic Depressive Association, Spirit Menders and peer counselors. These groups are generally nonprofessional, client-run and aimed at support and education. Occupational therapists are viewed as resources and mentors. Involvement with self-help groups has created an occupational therapy practice where therapists have a rich assortment of referral information and educational information about specific psychiatric diagnoses on hand.

A member of POTAC also represented occupational therapy on the state wide *Task Force on Families and Mental Illness*. This task force "is part of a project being conducted by the California Alliance for the Mentally Ill, and supported by the California Department of Mental Health (Special Legislative Program-AB 1278-1989). It is concerned primarily with pre-service training options for mental health professionals . . ." (Backer & Husted, 1991). As part of this project, the Occupational Therapy Department of San Jose State University began incorporating the family experience of mental illness into their curricula. Guest speakers from the local CAMI members are invited to speak in selected classes and their presentations are evaluated by students. The response by occupational therapy students has been overwhelmingly positive and specific evaluative data continues to be collected. Occupational therapy academic programs must take a leading role in preparing future occupational therapists for a rapidly changing mental health practice. To this end, the inclusion of the family perspective is one major component.

Occupational therapists who are members of POTAC are also involved with local mental health advisory boards, both on the institutional, and city and county level, as well as on the state level. A city or county mental health board is typically mandated by the state to advise boards of supervisors, directors of public health and directors of mental health regarding appropriate and meaningful mental health services. In San Francisco, a Community Advisory Board is mandated by a city ordinance to involve San Francisco's residents in the planning, evaluation and monitoring of psychiatric services for San Francisco General Hospital. POTAC recently participated in a very well received panel presentation to the San Francisco Mental Health Board on "The Use of the Arts in Therapy." The acting Director of Occupational Therapy at San Francisco General Hospital is the staff's link to the hospital advisory board. The group is seeking to form a partnership with the Mental Health Association which is another advocacy agency.

Another important area for therapists with a CCP and for POTAC members is lobbying state and federal legislators. POTAC is active in the AOTA government affairs network. Information from the *Action Line* publication is routinely disseminated at meetings and in newsletters. POTAC members are represented on the Occupational Therapy Association of California government affairs, third party reimbursement, practice, and ways and means committees. One POTAC member reviews all state legislation regarding mental health and routinely attends a group called the California Coalition for Mental Health. This group is a large, broad based mental health advocacy group representing one hundred and fifteen thousand members, consisting of mental health provider and administrative associations, consumers and family groups. Other members of POTAC are active in political activities associated with the Association of Ambulatory Behavioral Health (AABH), California Association of Social Rehabilitation Agencies (CASARA) and the International Association of Psychosocial Rehabilitation Services (IAPRS).

CONCLUSION

POTAC is committed to research, study groups, workshops and in-service education, as well as reallocating a greater proportion of the profession's resources from the institution to community-based services. These commitments are also clearly part of a CCP. The POTAC group includes occupational therapists who are also adult education instructors, private practitioners, consultants, case managers, home health therapists, academics, managers and grant writers. The City and County of San Francisco Community Mental Health Department has just accepted a grant proposal on Assertive Community Treatment that was solely authored by an occupational therapist. A local Mental Health Association recently hired an occupational therapist for the first time. POTAC's contribution and the possibilities for the future are endless. Both POTAC and the CCP model advocate lifelong learning, and empowerment for ourselves and our clients (CAOT, 1993). Both have a broad vision of the profession's potential. POTAC and CCP is a winning combination.

ACKNOWLEDGMENTS

The authors wish to acknowledge the many dedicated occupational therapists who continue to contribute to the efforts described in this paper. Among them are: Kim Aspelund, Eileen Auerbach, Pat Bascom, Beth Ching, Karen Diasio-Serrett, Maria Dilliard, Georgette Dufresne, Olivia Flores, Susan Lang, Ardie McDermott, Ruth McFadden Ramsey, Elizabeth Schwehm, Renais Winter.

REFERENCES

Backer, T. & Husted, J. (May, 1991). *Report of the First Annual Conference of the Task Force on Families and Mental Illness*. California Alliance for the Mentally Ill.
Bowen, R. (May, 1996). Practicing What We Preach. *OT Week*, 20-24.
Clark, C., Scott, E., Krupa, T. (1993). Involving clients in programme evaluation

and research: A new methodology for occupational therapy. *Canadian Journal of Occupational Therapy*, (*4*), 192-199.

Canadian Association of Occupational Therapists (1993). *Occupational therapy guidelines for client-centered mental health practice*. Canada: Minister of Supply and Services.

Lang, S., Kannenberg, K. & Brinson, M. (1992). *50 simple things you can do to promote occupational therapy in mental health*. American Occupational Therapy Association. Rockville, MD.

Law, M., Baptiste, S., Mill, J. (1995). Client-centred practice: What does it mean and does it make a difference? *Canadian Journal of Occupational Therapy*, *62*(5), 250-257.

Law, M., Baptiste, S., Carswell, A., McColl, M. A., Polatajko H., & Pollock, N. (1994). *Canadian occupational performance measure*. Toronto: CAOT Publications.

Peternelj-Taylor, C. & Hartley, V. (1993). Living with mental illness: Professional/family collaboration. *Journal of Psychosocial Nursing*, *3*(3), 23-28.

Pollock, N. (1993). Client-centered assessment. *American Journal of Occupational Therapy*. *47*(4), 298-301.

Tapper, B. (February, 1996). New opportunities for mental health OTs. *OT Week*, pp. 16-17.

Tewfik, D. (March, 1995). Mental health practitioners in New York take action. *OT Week*, p 12.

The New York Experience:
The Remodeling of Mental Health Practice

Diane Tewfik, MA, OTR
Pat Precin, MS, OTR

SUMMARY. In response to changes in health care delivery, a coalition of therapists in New York City mounted a campaign to network with peers on the local, state and national level to exchange information and resources. The Mental Health Task Force explored new models of practice such as psychiatric home care, developed alliances with consumers and monitored regulatory agencies and legislation. *[Article copies available for a fee from The Haworth Document Delivery Service: 1-800-342-9678. E-mail address: getinfo@haworthpressinc.com]*

The 1990's have generated significant challenges in New York State. Budget cuts and downsizing brought fear and uncertainty to health care workers. Managed care came slowly to New York City and preparation for its impact in many cases was inadequate. Facilities closed, departments disbanded and reorganized, all in an attempt to be cost-effective for the next health maintenance organiza-

Diane Tewfik is Assistant Professor and Fieldwork Coordinator, City University of New York and York College, Department of Health Sciences, Occupational Therapy Program, 94-20 Guy R. Brewer Boulevard, Jamaica, NY 11451.

Pat Precin is Assistant Director of Occupational Therapy, Recreational Therapy, and Creative Arts Therapy, St. Lukes & Roosevelt Hospital, Dual Diagnosis Program, Suite 6C, 411 West 114th Street, New York, NY 10025.

[Haworth co-indexing entry note]: "The New York Experience: The Remodeling of Mental Health Practice." Tewfik, Diane, and Pat Precin. Co-published simultaneously in *Occupational Therapy in Mental Health* (The Haworth Press, Inc.) Vol. 14, No. 1/2, 1998, pp. 45-53; and: *New Frontiers in Psychosocial Occupational Therapy* (ed: Anne Hiller Scott) The Haworth Press, Inc., 1998, pp. 45-53. Single or multiple copies of this article are available for a fee from The Haworth Document Delivery Service [1-800-342-9678, 9:00 a.m. - 5:00 p.m. (EST). E-mail address: getinfo@haworthpressinc.com].

tion (HMO). These changes took their toll on occupational therapy staffing patterns and student training.

In this atmosphere, the Metropolitan New York District (MNYD) of the New York State Occupational Therapy Association's (NY-SOTA) Mental Health Task Force was formed in March of 1995. Committed therapists pledged to arrest the decline of practice and to revitalize mental health occupational therapy by adapting new models and strategies of action. Three subgroups were formed to address strategic areas: marketing and managed care focusing on how to interface with network systems; cost-effective occupational therapy treatment models; and publicity and political action for occupational therapy services (Tewfik, 1995).

Networking with mental health representatives was implemented at all levels of the local, state, and national professional associations. Through formal and informal networks, information was quickly disseminated and vital issues regularly explored. Therapists, who often worked in isolation around downsizing and problems related to managed care, accessed new information and developed new strategies. The task force became an important source of professional socialization and support for its members. The task force was able to develop a new role for each, a role of empowerment. Many therapists had felt not only isolated, but also powerless in the face of new changes. Often it was heard from a member after sharing a problem, "I really need this group." Meetings were not only a time to dialogue but to actively develop a positive role in revitalizing the profession.

MARKETING

Exchanges with consumers took place, forging alliances to provide quality care and to better market mental health occupational therapy services. In meetings with the Alliance of the Mentally Ill/Friends and Advocates of the Mentally Ill (AMI/FAMI), task force members highlighted the importance and cost-effectiveness of occupational therapy services in mental health. A referral system was developed to help consumers gain access to local therapists. The Mental Health Task Force was also instrumental in providing feedback to the MNYD and NYSOTA boards, supporting the development of a consumer directory statewide.

A consumer friendly fact sheet, "Mental Health Occupational Therapy, What It Is and How It Works, A Guide for Consumers," was developed for the education of consumers, families, and their support systems (Carlson, 1995). A consumer advocate, Mary Auslander, MSW, Director of Recipient Affairs, New York State Office of Mental Health, provided invaluable assistance in critiquing this document from the consumers' perspective.

A serious commitment to consumer advocacy was demonstrated by both members of the task force and consumers during a workshop entitled, "Dialogue with Consumers" (Scott, 1996). The consumers made valuable suggestions requesting an understanding of the rationales behind intervention and supported the idea of "seamless" treatment. The consumer panelists also emphasized the need for therapeutic tasks to be relevant to them as individuals, and expressed an interest in ongoing work with therapists to advocate for continued quality treatment. Based on the recommendations of this consumer panel, the MNYD board formulated a goal for 1997/1998 to expand consumer interface with all committees.

COST-EFFECTIVE MODELS

With the closing of many state hospitals in New York, the task force felt that priority should be given to a new model of health care delivery that could have the highest growth potential. Treatment models were examined and mental health home health care emerged as an innovative paradigm. Psychiatric home care is often the most cost-effective intervention and also offers a profound partnership involving client, family, practitioner, and the entire therapy network (AABH, 1995).

Occupational therapy is recognized by the Health Care Financing Administration (HCFA, 1989), as a reimbursable Medicare service for homebound patients diagnosed with a psychiatric illness. However, in New York City, it was found that only a handful of occupational therapists were engaged in mental health home care. Upon further inquiry, home health care agencies expressed reluctance about beginning such a service, although Visiting Nurse Service

(VNS) agencies (Cooper & Johnson, 1996; Earle-Grimes & Taegder, 1993) in other states have developed successful programs. Rehabilitation directors indicated that documentation was a primary factor in their reluctance to include mental health occupational therapy in their services. The guidelines for mental health home care are the same as those for general occupational therapy. They require that the patient needs skilled therapy services that can only be provided by an occupational therapist and that the patient be homebound (Menosky, 1995). Agencies contacted were skeptical that significant progress could be documented over a limited time frame (8-9 weeks) and on a week to week basis, which is required for Medicare reimbursement.

The task force at present is examining different documentation models, including Dombrowski (1990; 1996) and Allen's Cognitive Levels (ACL) (Allen, Earhart, & Blue, 1992; Allen, Blue, & Earhart, 1995). The ACL has been used effectively in several psychiatric home health care programs (Cooper & Johnson, 1996; Earle-Grimes & Taegder, 1993). Our future plans include presentations to educate potential referral systems on the role of occupational therapy in mental health home care.

The Program for Assertive Community Treatment/Assertive Community Treatment (PACT/ACT) was also examined. The comprehensive PACT model was pioneered in Madison, Wisconsin, for the treatment and rehabilitation services of persons with severe mental illness. Most ACT teams provide 24 hour a day coverage, with home-based interventions, pragmatic outcome-oriented treatment, and individualized goals as key elements in this model (Lachance & Santos, 1995; Santos, Henggeler, Burns, Arana, & Meisler, 1995). One study indicated that ACT clients were hospitalized about half as often as clients in standard services and were also less likely to be without a permanent residence (Essock, & Kontos, 1995).

Six of the eleven ACT teams in New York City were contacted, but none employed occupational therapists. One agency did state that they had a line for either an occupational therapist or a vocational counselor but chose a vocational counselor because of the "vocational component." This led the task force to conclude that education about occupational therapy roles and services is critical. Occupational therapists must also be educated as to their potential in community mental health, for example, acting as consultants to ACT teams, assessing and defining clinical interventions relevant to community living and employment, and providing supervision to students working in this model, further opening up the realm of services in community mental health (Schindler, & Swarbrick, 1995).

REGULATION OF MANAGED CARE NETWORKS

The regulation of managed care networks was also investigated. Initially there were no regulatory systems in place, however, in 1994 the Joint Commission on Accreditation of Healthcare Organizations (JCAHO) developed their first set of standards specifically for managed care networks (JCAHO, 1994a). The accreditation services were then voluntary. Subsequently, eight states have enacted legislation for mandatory regulation: Florida, Indiana, Kansas, Oklahoma, Nevada, South Carolina, Texas, and Washington and eleven other states have requested mandatory regulation (JCAHO, 1996a). Networks with accreditation have the opportunity to reduce cost, improve quality, and demonstrate accountability, all critical elements for long term success in a fluctuating health care marketplace, as the results of each network's evaluation are published for review.

We participated in a field review of the *1994 Standards for Health Care Networks* (JCAHO, 1994b). The one hundred thirty page manuscript was very general and addressed many areas of central structure, but usually included a loophole with the ultimate decision making power given to the managed care network itself, thus undermining the purpose of having specific standards for adherence.

The appendix dealing with *Standards for the Mentally Ill, Chemically Dependent, Mental Retardation and Developmental Disabilities* (JCAHO, 1994b) had several critical omissions. There was no mention of the need to insure the use of appropriate, licensed professionals in patient assessment and treatment. Physical therapy and nursing were included in the document, but occupational therapy was not mentioned. This was a marked omission in comparison to the 1995 JCAHO hospital standards which included numerous references to occupational therapy (Scalenger, 1995). Furthermore, the document did not include diagnostic, medical and functional guidelines. There was no section addressing the treatment of the mentally ill or substance abuse, although the treatment section for developmental disabilities and mental retardation was well developed. Self care was addressed superficially, with the potential for decreased quality of care. The areas of health promotion and disease prevention were underdeveloped with no mention of occupational therapy.

The task group submitted proposed revisions in June, 1995. A year later the revised *1996 Comprehensive Accreditation Manual for Health Care Networks* by JCAHO (1996b) was published. Upon review, it was found that none of our recommendations had been incorporated. Through subsequent inquiry with AOTA, we learned that the Coalition of Rehabilitative Therapy Organization (CRTO), where occupational therapy has representation, does not have a seat on the Network Professional and Technical Advisory Committee (PTAC) which provides further input on such documents. This means that information about networks (such as our review) may have stopped in midstream. Based on our concern to actively monitor JCAHO regulations, we are now receiving the JCAHO newsletter and are vigilantly reviewing developments in this area.

Several additional projects have emerged from this review process: review of standards for the National Committee on Quality Assurance (NCQA) and the Association of Ambulatory Behavioral Health Care (AABHC), which is currently writing standards for psychiatric home care; contact with other organizations who are reviewing and writing standards such as the National Association of State and Mental Health Directors; and lobbying for the mandatory regulation of health care networks in New York State.

POLITICAL ACTION

The Legislative and Government Relations Coordinator for NY-SOTA, Jeffrey Tomlinson, focused on a number of legislative issues including managed care regulation. During 1996, NYSOTA actively participated in a large coalition of health care providers and consumers to fight for reasonable managed care practices. The coalition facilitated the passage of a comprehensive bill in the legislature prohibiting exclusion of any type of licensed provider and requiring the use of either physicians or occupational therapy practitioners within the same specialty to perform utilization reviews of occupational therapy services.

The state budget process was monitored and occupational therapy practitioners were alerted to major cuts of 25% proposed in the mental health budget. A coalition of therapists, providers and consumers lobbied in the State Capitol to reduce cuts to 12%. Lobbying pressure also protected the State's Community Mental Health Reinvestments Act directing money saved by closing down state operated inpatient units, toward expanding community services. The legislative committee is continuously monitoring key legislation in the State.

GOALS FOR THE FUTURE

The MNYD Mental Health Task Force is looking forward to another active year and has formulated critical goals for 1998. Our initiatives include goals to: increase consumer related activities; develop models for mental health home care; network with and educate consumers, political and business groups; increase marketing of occupational therapy; disseminate information through local, state, and national networking; and explore computer resources. To facilitate these goals we have co-authored (Scott, Swarbrick, Tewfik & Precin, 1997) with Peggy Swarbrick of the New Jersey Network on Wellness a grant funded by CSAP (Committee of State Association Presidents of AOTA); which will create an on-line resource through AOTA and NYSOTA for a "Clearinghouse for Consumer Centered Community OT Models in Mental Health and Physical Disabilities." The focus of the New York group is a small part of what the entire profession needs to achieve. We urge all to join their local coalition to support this vital mission. Together we can remodel and revitalize mental health occupational therapy practice.

ACKNOWLEDGMENTS

The authors would like to gratefully acknowledge Anne Hiller Scott for her thoughtful review and feedback and for her leadership in the task force, as well as the other task force leaders including Cheryl King, Suzanne White, Hanna Diamond, Joan Feder and Sheri Wadler. We also gratefully recognize the following therapists for their contributions: Tina Barth, Paulette Bell, Ann Burkhardt, Danielle Butin, Jodi Carlson, Alisa Chazani, Elinor Cohen, Leora Cohen, Lynn Dombrowski, Gloria Graham, Sue Himmelbauer, Carlotta Kip, Stanley Shing-Kung Li, Ruth Meiers, Ruth Meyers, Liza Ness, Marian Kavanaugh Scheinholtz, Rose Solomon, Virginia Stoffel, Peggy Swarbrick, Ellen Taira, Jeffrey Tomlinson, and Aileen Yamaguchi. We extend sincere thanks to our consumer advisors: Mary Auslander, Justine Hopper, and Dave Schneider.

REFERENCES

Allen, C., Earhart, C., & Blue, T. (1992). *Occupational therapy treatment goals for the physically and cognitively disabled*. Rockville, MD: American Occupational Therapy Association.

Allen, C., Blue, T., & Earhart, C. (1995). *Understanding cognitive performance modes*. Ormond Beach, FL: Allen Conferences, Inc.

The Association for Ambulatory Behavioral Health Care. (1995). *Inside AABH: Psychiatric home care: The next ambulatory wave?* (1995). (pp. 12-13). Fairfax, VA.

Carlson, J. (1995). *Mental health occupational therapy and private practice*. Speech given at the New York State Occupational Therapy Conference, NY.

Cooper, R., & Johnson, A. T. (1996, April). *Mental health programming within a home care agency*. Speech at the 76th Annual American Occupational Therapy Conference in Chicago, IL.

Dombrowski, L. B. (1990). *Functional needs assessment. Program for chronic psychiatric patients*. San Antonio, TX: Therapy Skill Builders.

Dombrowski, L. B., & Kane, M. A. (1996). *Functional needs assessment treatment guide*. San Antonio, TX: Therapy Skill Builders.

Earle-Grimes, G., & Taegder, L. (1993, June). *Psychiatric home health in the 90's*. Speech at the 73rd Annual American Occupational Therapy Association Conference in Seattle, WA.

Essock, S. M., & Kontos, N. (1995, July). Implementing assertive community treatment teams. *Psychiatric Services, 46*(7): 679-83.

Health Care Financing Administration. (1989). *Health insurance manual, 11*, (Sections 204.1 and 205.2). Washington, DC: US Government Printing Office.

JCAHO. (1994a). *Accreditation manual for health care networks*. Oakbrook, IL: Joint Commission on Accreditation of Healthcare Organizations.

JCAHO. (1994b). *Revised appendixes to the 1994 accreditation manual for health care networks*. Oakbrook, IL.: Joint Commission on Accreditation of Healthcare Organizations.

JCAHO. (1996a). *Network news*. Issue two, 1-2. Oakbrook, IL: Joint Commission on Accreditation of Healthcare Organizations.

JCAHO. (1996b). *Comprehensive accreditation manual for health care networks*. Oakbrook, IL.: Joint Commission on Accreditation of Healthcare Organizations.

Lachance, K. R. & Santos, A. B. (1995, June). Modifying the PACT model: Preserving critical elements. *Psychiatric Services, 46*(6): 601-4.

Menosky, J. (1995). Mental health services in the home health setting: Special considerations. In, *Guidelines for occupational therapy practice in home health* (pp. 43-54). Bethesda, MD: American Occupational Therapy Association, Inc.

Santos, A. B., Henggeler, S. W., Burns, B. J., Arana, G. W., & Meisler, N. (1995, August). Research on field-based services: Models for reform in the delivery of mental health care to populations with complex clinical problems. *American Journal of Psychiatry, 152*(8): 1111-23.

Scalenger, R. (April 11, 1995). *The Joint Commission's (JCAHO'S) new hospital standards.* Speech at the AOTA's 1995 Annual Conference, Denver, CO.

Schindler, V. & Swarbrick, P. (1995). *The role of occupational therapy on a PACT team.* Unpublished manuscript.

Scott, A. H. (May, 1996). Dialogue with consumers. *MNYD Memo,* pp. 10-11.

Scott, A. H., Swarbrick, P., Tewfik, D. & Precin, P. (1997). CSAP Incentive Award Application, 1997. *A Clearinghouse for Consumer Centered Community Models in Mental Health and Physical Disabilities.*

Tewfik, D. (1995, March 27). Mental health practitioners in New York take action. *OT Week,* 11-12.

Dialogue with Consumers

Anne Hiller Scott, PhD, OTR, FAOTA

Setting: Metropolitan New York District of New York State Occupational Therapy Association, Mental Health Special Interest Group Meeting–February 27, 1996

Audience: Occupational Therapists, occupational therapy students

Purpose: To have an exchange at the "grass roots" level with consumers of psychiatric services

Topic: Dialogue with Consumers

Panelists: Cheryl King, MA, OTR, CRC, Moderator/coordinator of the panel

Joan Feder, MA, OTR, CRC, Coordinator of an Intensive Psychiatric Rehabilitation Program

Justine Hopper, consumer and peer advocate at Community Access

Dave Schneider, consumer and co-editor of *Choices–Newsletter for the Self Help Movement*

Mary Auslander, MSW, New York State Office of Mental Hygiene, Office of Recipient Affairs

DISCUSSION

As consumer advocate, Mary Auslander surveyed the audience noting that she was unaware of who were consumers and who were

Anne Hiller Scott is Director, Division of Occupational Therapy, School of Health Professions, Long Island University-Brooklyn Campus, 1 University Plaza, Brooklyn, NY 11201.

[Haworth co-indexing entry note]: "Dialogue with Consumers." Scott, Anne Hiller. Co-published simultaneously in *Occupational Therapy in Mental Health* (The Haworth Press, Inc.) Vol. 14, No. 1/2, 1998, pp. 55-56; and: *New Frontiers in Psychosocial Occupational Therapy* (ed: Anne Hiller Scott) The Haworth Press, Inc., 1998, pp. 55-56. Single or multiple copies of this article are available for a fee from The Haworth Document Delivery Service [1-800-342-9678, 9:00 a.m. - 5:00 p.m. (EST). E-mail address: getinfo@haworthpressinc.com].

providers. She commented that if we were really working towards inclusion "There should be a 50/50 mix of consumers and providers at the table."

How many of us could meet this challenge? The desire to engage with consumers in meaningful exchange had prompted our local group to assemble this panel and this was obviously just the beginning. How do any of us work with individual service recipients to bridge the patient/therapist gap and transcend traditional professional boundaries to support common causes? Many of us are still in the process of searching for effective methods and vehicles. This panel riveted us in our search for a focus–it became clear that on a local level we needed to develop relationships with consumer groups and this became a pivotal objective for the upcoming year for the local Metropolitan New York District board and also for the state board of the New York State Occupational Therapy Association.

In all areas of practice the consumer's voice is compelling and must be heard. This compilation of articles emerged from the panelists who participated in the "Dialogue with Consumers." In the new frontiers of mental health practice, consumers have moved from the backwards to the front lines. Each of the consumers on this panel agreed to make their voices heard to an even broader audience through this publication.

In this series of articles we will feature Justine Hopper, a consumer with multiple physical disabilities, who found her experience with mental illness far more stigmatizing. Joan Feder will present a model program of empowerment for consumers seeking vocational rehabilitation. In another article, Mary Auslander will speak to both sides of the issue from her dual perspective as a consumer and a provider. David Schneider will address the ADA (Americans with Disabilities Act) as it relates to mental illness and disclosure.

It is hoped that through the dialogue with consumers that follows, each of us will be moved to consider how we can rise to the challenge of bringing consumers to the table in the true spirit of inclusion, forging meaningful alliances that will promote the quality of care that we all seek.

Out of the Ashes

Justine B. Hopper

SUMMARY. From the aftermath of a failed suicide attempt, a consumer describes her painful journey through a long course of psychosocial rehabilitation in a day treatment program, culminating in the cherished goal of employment. As an individual with multiple disabilities, her past experience with occupational therapy in physical rehabilitation only addressed the presenting body part, not the whole person. Her feelings and need to learn emotional coping skills were not acknowledged until her desperate call for help through an overdose. In the process of becoming whole, she deals with the new stigma of an even more disabling label–mental illness. *[Article copies available for a fee from The Haworth Document Delivery Service: 1-800-342-9678. E-mail address: getinfo@haworthpressinc.com]*

I was worthless, and alone. I despaired. I had one choice. I would take my life. It was the second attempt in two years, the third time in nine. This time was like the others in method and reason. Only now it was planned with indifference. I had taken a combination of Advil and Tylenol, because I knew no other way of coping with my problems. I had overdue bills. I had gone through frequent evaluations for a vocational training program that might have led me to a job. But the prospects of getting one, a paying job, that is, were nil. I was also overwhelmed with volunteer work I had been doing for an organization I had been involved with for many years. I was

---

Justine B. Hopper is Peer Specialist, Community Access, 3rd Floor, 666 Broadway, New York, NY 10012.

[Haworth co-indexing entry note]: "Out of the Ashes." Hopper, Justine B. Co-published simultaneously in *Occupational Therapy in Mental Health* (The Haworth Press, Inc.) Vol. 14, No. 1/2, 1998, pp. 57-65; and: *New Frontiers in Psychosocial Occupational Therapy* (ed: Anne Hiller Scott) The Haworth Press, Inc., 1998, pp. 57-65. Single or multiple copies of this article are available for a fee from The Haworth Document Delivery Service [1-800-342-9678, 9:00 a.m. - 5:00 p.m. (EST). E-mail address: getinfo@haworthpressinc.com].

expected, that very morning, to be on a train bound for Connecticut to deliver work (not done at all), and to visit friends who were part of this organization. These concerns were too much for me.

I thought no one would understand the pain and anguish I was feeling. I could have gone to my family, friends or my psychiatrist for help, but I trusted no one. I feared I would be chastised instead of helped. I thought I had failed. I believed that if anyone found out about my imperfections they would think I was not responsible for my own needs. I would feel even more guilty, more ashamed and more worthless because I would always need help. I thought that suicide was the only alternative to a lifetime of humiliation.

Much to my chagrin, I had failed again. The pills didn't work. I was still alive some six hours later. Instead of being dead, I felt sick. I only went for help to relieve the nausea I felt. I called my parents not knowing, or caring about, how they would feel. I showed no remorse for my actions. I was indifferent to their feelings and numb to my own. I was unaware of the possible result of my actions. My parents drove me to the hospital. I remember while fishing for the seat belt in front of my Dad's car, my Dad asking, "Why are you looking for a seat belt to protect yourself from a bang on the head when you just tried to kill yourself?" This question did not faze me, nor did the consequences that were yet to follow.

The choice I had made on March 28, 1993, changed my life. I was admitted that night to the Psychiatric Unit at NYU Medical Center. My awareness of that first night in the hospital is vague, but I still remember how I felt. I felt like a convicted criminal. Although I was a patient, I was treated like a prisoner. I did something wrong and was being punished for it. Yes, my suicide attempt was wrong. There were other rational choices I could have made. Why then was I being punished for being sick? My diagnosis was clinical depression. My sentence was thirty days. Now, I had not only to face a month in "jail," a devastated family and friends, but also another label!

TO BE PHYSICALLY DISABLED . . .

Congenital toxoplasmosis had left me with lateral brain damage, and a scarred retina. As a result, I have cerebral palsy on my left side, a history of seizures, only peripheral vision in my right eye, and just light perception in my left. I have adapted to these disabilities logistically. My feelings of anger, resentment and frustration regarding them, however, were masked by my determination to overcome them in order to survive in a "normal" world.

My determination to be "mainstreamed" into the "normal" world was an ongoing and often self defeating goal. I also wanted to be mainstreamed into the world of my disabled peers as well. As much as I tried, I was never accepted by my disabled peers. I stood out as being different. I was rejected for having one disability too many. I belonged nowhere.

. . . TO BE A MENTAL PATIENT

I felt fearful and empty as I awoke from a sleepless night in NYU Medical Center to start my first day as a mental patient. My only exposure to "real" mental patients was in books, movies and T.V. I never knew anyone who was diagnosed "crazy," and I certainly did not think I would be one of them! My admission to NYU Medical Center was my official initiation into the mental health care system.

Even though I had been in therapy on and off for nine years, I had no idea of what it really meant to be a mental patient. The therapy I received was merely a Band-Aid for the immediate problem. Once the problem was resolved, my feelings would lay dormant only to crop up again later.

My hospitalization gave me a bitter taste of the stigma of the mentally ill. Stigma was not new to me as a multiply disabled person. I was often mistaken as being retarded because of my awkward gait and the involuntary movement of my eyes. Since I travel around fairly well, friends and even professionals seemed to have difficulty understanding why I don't recognize them and say "Hello." My needs even became a taboo to physical and occupational therapists. I was trained in visual mobility, vocational skills and activities in daily living skills. I was never considered by any agency as a package deal. The specialty of the occupational therapist would determine which part of my body (eyes or right hand) I would take with me. The stigma of being multiply disabled was far easier to swallow than being a mentally ill patient. I was to possess a feeling of vulnerability and a helplessness that would forever leave an indelible mark on my mind and heart.

MEDS OF THE UNDEAD

When I was admitted to NYU Medical Center, the attending psychiatrist immediately put me on 30 mg. of Prozac three times a day for the depression and 5 mg. of Haldol twice a day to organize my thoughts. Although I had never heard of, let alone taken, this medication before, I expected to be given something to help me feel better. Since I had been taking different types of medication for seizures in the past with minor side effects, I thought I had no reason to question the expertise of my doctor.

As the days wore on, I started having problems. I had blurred vision and loss in concentration. I was restless and tired. I had trouble sleeping when it was time to sleep and was on the nod when I wanted to be awake and alert. I had severe spasms in my neck and in an already spastic left arm and leg. The hangover I experienced only got worse as the days went on. I felt like one of Dracula's "undead." I was not dead, but I was not alive either. These symptoms affected my functioning, but I went on the best I could. After the first week and a half, I started complaining to the staff. My voice was ignored. I was told to concentrate on something else. When my family members saw what was happening to me, they advocated for me. They intervened and got the resident on call to examine me. The doctor prescribed Cogentin to help with some of the side effects.

I realized for the first time that the stigma of a person whose disabilities are visibly obvious was different from the stigma I was now experiencing as a mental patient with no visible disability. This was hard ball. There were no rules. There was no respect, only fear.

Instead of my initial fear that a patient would get out of hand and hurt me, I spent the rest of my time at NYU fearing my attending psychiatrist. The doctor explained to me that the purpose of the medication was to prevent me from trying to kill myself again. I tried to explain, with support from my family, that I felt I was being over medicated not to prevent another suicide attempt, but to keep me from causing trouble. I also stated that my family's concern for me was only listened to in order to shut them up. Once I was informed of my right to refuse medication, I refused to take the Prozac which, for me, had bad side effects. The daily psychotherapy group and my socializing with my peers was the nourishment I needed to get me through my stay. I had found for the first time in my life, a safe place to talk about my feelings, past and present. Their empathy and support enabled me to trust others. The seeds for recovery were planted but I was not ready. I couldn't wait to get out and pick up my life where I had left off.

DAY TREATMENT

Much to my dismay, this was not to be the case. Before I was discharged from NYU it was suggested by the on-unit social worker that I attend a "Continuing Day Treatment Program (CDTP)." The unit staff and my family agreed. I reluctantly agreed to go for an interview.

I felt like a lamb led to slaughter when I walked into the room for the interview, I was intimidated by the thirty people I saw that were ready to tear me apart with their questions. This treatment team consisted of doctors, nurses, social workers and occupational therapists, all of whom would play an important role in my recovery. Since I could not see the expressions on their faces, I misread the concern in their voices as being stern. I wanted to escape from this lion's den before I was eaten alive. I was especially resentful when I was informed that I could not drink any more. I am not an alcoholic, but I did use it as a self medicator when I was depressed. I was also horrified that I had to talk about my feelings with people I did not know. I knew, however, that I had to do something. When I was accepted into the program, I resigned myself to give it a try. I started St. Vincent's CDTP on April 29, 1993, the day after I was discharged from NYU.

CULTURE SHOCK

I experienced a real culture shock when I started the CDTP program at St. Vincent's. The patients who attended the Day Program came from different economic classes, educational backgrounds, religions and sexual orientations. They also represented different psychiatric disabilities. As a native New Yorker, I was used to going to school and socializing with people from economic, educational and religious backgrounds different from my own. I was not, however, used to being around people of different sexual orientations. This was only part of the culture shock.

Whenever I received occupational therapy in the past, I was never encouraged to talk about anything other than learning the task at hand. I was never taught how to cope emotionally with my disabilities. I believed that if any service provider found out about my psychiatric history I would lose my apartment, my benefits and be banned from any program I was in. I was forced for the first time at St. Vincent's CDTP to talk about my feelings. I was horrified!

Eventually, I settled in and was ready to work. The three years that I spent at St. Vincent's CDTP program were the hardest years of my life. Not one academic course I had taken was as hard as this one. I was constantly opening up wounds that had healed and old ones that had not healed at all. I discovered through therapy that I needed to change my patterns in thinking and expressing my feelings. I found that I had never allowed myself to be angry at anything, especially my disabilities. I was raised to believe that they were a part of me, that I should go on in spite of them. I should play the hand I was dealt. I never knew it was O.K. to be angry. I learned with the help of the staff and my peers at St. Vincent's, how to express this anger in a controlled manner.

LIKE A FULL TIME JOB

The day program gave structure to my day for the first time, a reason to get up in the morning. I looked on it as a job. For the first year and a half, I was enrolled in fifteen groups. I came in five days a week, for five hours a day. These groups varied in both subject and substance. "Family Studies," and "Human Relations" taught me how to communicate better with others. In "Affective Disorders" I learned about the different types of psychiatric illnesses and the different medications and their side effects. The socialization groups I participated in were "Performance Group," "Drama" and "Leisure." I was also required to take "Clean and Sober" to help me cope with my "drinking problem." All of the groups I participated in were designed to help me integrate into the community and become a "whole person" again. For my part however, this idea of integrating me as a whole person was new.

The groups I had taken in the first year and a half were a necessary foundation for other groups to follow. When the team felt I was ready, I started "Psychotherapy" and "Cognitive Therapy." These groups gave me the tools I needed to cope with my feelings and to change distortions in my thinking.

In "Cognitive Therapy," I learned through reading, role playing and experimentation, that my feelings are neither right nor wrong. I also learned that there are more than two sides to a problem. I immersed myself in this group and learned a great deal.

"Psychotherapy" had a different focus altogether. The members of the group, including the Occupational Therapist, worked as a team in order to interact, discuss and solve individuals' problems. I was respected and accepted as a peer, more than any other group I was in. This was where I bared my soul, my private thoughts and feelings. My body was merely a storage container. I was not "mainstreamed." I was normal!

In addition to groups, I had bi-weekly meetings with my case manager and my doctor. I discussed specific problems that I could not discuss in regular groups. My therapy was not limited to learning how to cope with my own feelings, problems and actions. Family meetings played a major role in my therapy. I found out through these meetings how truly loved I am. Therapy was more painful for my family than it was for me. Yet, they came and participated because they wanted to do everything they could to help me. Everything from my keeping secret my suicide attempts to dispelling my lifelong feeling that my three brothers and my sister resented me because of the extra attention I got growing up. It all came out during these meetings. Unlike the first meeting we had at NYU, where everything I wanted to say was fair game, family members were not obligated to bring everything up. The rights of everyone were respected during the meetings at St. Vincent's. My relationship with my family has changed as a result. I am no longer afraid to be honest or direct. I am now able to accept the same thing from them.

Three of the groups I was in, "Gazette," "Pre Voc" and "Peer Advocacy," were to make an important impact on my future as a person and a "consumer." "Gazette" is the name of the CDTP's in-house newspaper. The group met four times a week. The immediate goal of the group was to put together a monthly newspaper consisting of poetry, short stories, consumer news and editorials. This group was the prerequisite to "Pre Voc," which focused on helping patients get ready to go to work or go to school. "Peer Advocacy" set up the agenda for the weekly community meeting. While writing for the "Gazette," brushing up on computer skills in "Pre Voc," and learning how to advocate for my fellow peers in "Peer Advocacy," I began to find my self-esteem which had been buried.

FINDING LIFE'S PURPOSE

On a Wednesday in October 1994, the occupational therapy leader in Pre Voc announced that there was going to be a meeting the next night to inform consumers of a new "Peer Specialist" training program. She thought that it would be great if I attended. I went with much reservation. I had been to these meetings before and nothing ever came of them. To my surprise, I was wrong.

The room was filled with twenty prospective peer specialist trainees. The organization that was to sponsor the program had five presenters. The first presenter talked about how the training program was to be run. He said that there would be a hundred hours in training ranging from counseling skills to AIDS awareness. Then he said, there would be a three to six month internship. I was sold immediately, but needed to ask him if I would be permitted to sign up because of my other disabilities, specifically my vision.

I discovered I had no need to worry. His response was genuine. He said that my having other disabilities would not be a problem. I don't know what it was, but a connection was made between us. It was one that often takes years of knowing someone to make. I sent in my request for an interview the next day. I was interviewed by the presenter and his right hand man in November. I received my acceptance letter for the program on Christmas Eve. It was a magnificent Christmas present. My dream of finding some direction in my life was coming true.

After going through the hundred hours of training, I interned at Community Access, in transitional housing. The training was invaluable and the internship solidified it. I was employed by Community Access in January of this year, 1996, a year after I entered the program. My long search for purpose in my life was realized. My experiences as a multiple disabled person had become assets.

In the changing field of mental health, it is disturbing to me, now a consumer, to find that money seems more important to some providers than caring for the people they serve. My salary check gives me the dignity I never had, but more importantly, helping people, the joy I've never known before. Something worthwhile came out of my brokenness. Now, the nightmare of NYU seems worth it, I was in the right place at the right time.

An Ex-Patient/Practitioner's Comments on Professional- and Consumerisms, with Poetry

Mary W. Auslander, MSW

SUMMARY. This article, more like a stream of consciousness or conversation, touches on a personal story and leads to a clinical/political stance. It seeks to convey some of the difficulties in the field's quest to practice "consumerism," the inclusion of mental health service recipients and ex-patients in all aspects of the mental health system. It tells part of the author's story as an ex-patient who has professionalized in the field, and offers readers the chance to ponder their roles relative to the recent phenomenon of asking consumers to participate. It concludes with poetry meant to be read as a letter to mental health workers from a composite client who seeks their support. *[Article copies available for a fee from The Haworth Document Delivery Service: 1-800-342-9678. E-mail address: getinfo@haworthpressinc.com]*

Anne Sexton, a Pulitzer Prize-winning poet, an ex-patient and abuse survivor, was once quoted as saying that she approached a very difficult poem by telling herself it was too hard to write, daring

Mary W. Auslander is former Recipient Affairs Specialist for the New York State Office of Mental Health in New York City. She is now a consultant and speaker, currently working with the National Empowerment Center, Box 230, East Dennis, MA 02641, and the Center for Mental Health Services.

[Haworth co-indexing entry note]: "An Ex-Patient/Practitioner's Comments on Professional- and Consumerisms, with Poetry." Auslander, Mary W. Co-published simultaneously in *Occupational Therapy in Mental Health* (The Haworth Press, Inc.) Vol. 14, No. 1/2, 1998, pp. 67-76; and: *New Frontiers in Psychosocial Occupational Therapy* (ed: Anne Hiller Scott) The Haworth Press, Inc., 1998, pp. 67-76. Single or multiple copies of this article are available for a fee from The Haworth Document Delivery Service [1-800-342-9678, 9:00 a.m. - 5:00 p.m. (EST). E-mail address: getinfo@haworthpressinc.com].

herself to surmount the task. Since being asked to write for the book, I recalled and tried her ploy, and then had to consider why it didn't work.

Aside from the historical fact that I generally face the prospect of writing with a period of semi-paralysis, I pondered if this time it related to being asked as an "expert" on matters of consumerism: how to include them, how to better understand their points of view, how to–what, remember that they are no different? From whom? You? Well, then, no different from me! But I have a history! Us and them . . . again? What do we mean by "consumer?" What do we mean by "inclusion?" Where have we been in the field if not heeding the "consumer!?"

How novel is this idea, that "we" would want the clients themselves to be involved in what is supposed to be a set of tools for them to use as they wish in their own lives? Is this too radical a translation of the fields claiming professionalism in mental health? Is it dreaming to envision people who've lived through psychiatric labeling and treatment as the theorists and program designers in the field? Am I delusional to think that people choose the field to be partners in healing rather than perpetrators of theory and enforcers of the social norm?

My mind was awash in this recurring stream of questions I have about the "therapies," what professionals are doing and how they are engaged with those called patients or more recently, consumers. I realized that I began to think in the generalizations and extremes I ask others not to–a sure sign of my anxiety around the subject. I welcome and dread being asked about involving consumers, who they are, what they have to offer, and why you ought to consider them the experts on a daily basis. The whole business is fraught with difficulties anew, such as having to consider what it means to be invited to the table at this time, and what happens if the power really begins to become equalized. (So far the latter presents no problem: consumers seldom get paid or credit as consultants, even when serving as key members of committees and task forces; their independent programs receive less than half of one percent of all funding in the field.)

I sought to answer myself in part when I produced my master's thesis for a degree in social work; "Voices from the Ex-patient

Movement: Psychiatric Survivors Unite and Heal" (Auslander, 1990) was one way to find out why those voices united while I avoided them through the years following my last hospitalization (the sixth in nine years). I had already stepped gingerly near the subject, doing undergraduate research on the family movement and on stigma. If I avoided my fellow-labeled folks, what of mental health professionals without psychiatric histories? How could they want to associate with the very people they wanted to "help" and with whom they had been largely trained to keep a very strict boundary?

I learned from my thesis subjects that the term mental patient is considered a more honest reflection of many persons' histories in contrast to "consumer." "Consumers" choose; no one chooses a psychiatric label and many are often forced into treatment, thus being made into mental patients. Since doing my thesis I continued to dance around the world of C/S/Xs (consumers/survivors/ex-patients–this is the term used by the National Empowerment Center and many leaders in the C/S/X movement). Recently, I leaped away from my deepest involvement with C/S/Xs and the bureaucracy mandated with responsibility for their services. Yet, I'm aware that being part of the C/S/X movement is the most singularly important influence on my identity and heart since being called (and made) a mental patient.

So why do I dance instead of steady myself in firm alignment with my like-kind? And I wonder, are occupational therapists, and other mental health professionals proud of their affiliation? Are they more proud of the boundaries they keep than the connections they make? Do they know why they are there? If not, why not? These seem the most basic questions about our callings, and this opportunity to reflect finds me hopeful that you will accompany me in reevaluating what may seem too obvious to consider.

If you want something instructive–such as "seven ways to include consumers in your program planning"–I won't let you down, but refer you to the good news of resources constructed by people who have been labeled mentally ill, whom you can learn from and support by directly seeking, and often paying for, their materials and ideas. In particular, you can call (as soon as you finish reading this) for the catalogue and newsletters of the National Empowerment Center (NEC).* Unlike the materials from NEC, some may find this too abstract. Yet we know the most valid way for real understanding to grow (as we often advise clients) is to gather our own resources and individualize the use of them. Beyond this I can only share some of my story and ideas in hope that you can extract meaning for yourself in your practice.

During my twenties I was hospitalized six times within nine years. Most of these admissions, coerced voluntary and involuntary, set me far back in my development, leaving me with many more complications and medications than I started with. When I realized I could not continue to let this occur (a crucial moment indeed), my recovery led me back to school; working my way through became my alternative institutionalization. I achieved a B.A. (Columbia) in 1988 and completed my master's degree in clinical social work in 1990. Like the period encompassing the hospitalizations, this too was a nine-year struggle, but infinitely more healing and rewarding. For more than four years, I deliberately sought direct clinical work in mental health settings, from out-patient adult in the South Bronx to residential for adolescents. I still believed I could help from within and do things differently from what I'd experienced.

My dual identity as an ex-patient and social worker became more of a burden as I went along, particularly because I'd finally found the movement of ex-patients, qualitatively studied their views, and lived with their–our–stories throbbing in the background of every team meeting where "cases" were discussed. I was acutely aware that I was working as a consenting part of a system where I found barriers to doing things differently in every direction, including within myself. I began to wonder if ending up there as a worker constituted another diagnosis.

Considering my peers' histories, I saw clearly that whether by "mis-diagnosis" or medications given injudiciously, whether by dehumanizing rituals that are routine in psychiatric wards and clin-

---

*The National Empowerment Center founded, directed and staffed by ex-patients, and funded by the Center for Mental Health Services, exists to promote recovery, empowerment, hope and healing through education, training, and mutual support. It is located at 20 Ballard Road, Lawrence, MA 01843-1018, and can be reached at 1-800-POWER 2 U.

ics, or by having one's judgment questioned in every interview with a mental health professional, we had all been hurt in the process of "being helped," even when we also had been helped. I began to despair of ever making a difference in the system, for to avoid its demands would be dishonest one way or another, either to authority or to clients. After all, the most basic premise for being seen in clinics and wards *is* being diagnosed, and often designated dangerous to self or others–an unquestioned criteria that hurts beyond words. Daily I wondered how I could "comply" with categorizing and labeling people "for their own good," or at least so that they could receive some sort of service. I found no answer, but, at last, hope.

Hope took the form of being told about an ex-patient who had gone so far as to become a psychiatrist in order to work in the field that had hurt him. Dan Fisher, currently the director of the National Empowerment Center and medical director at a community mental health clinic, had become well aware that other "consumer/practitioners" were out there who were struggling to keep their integrity along with their hard-won "sanity" while working in a very crazy field. He convened a meeting where I met people in the New York State Office of Mental Health (NYSOMH) who were coordinating a series of dialogues between psychiatrists in key positions and ex-patients, many of whom had become practitioners in the field (Blanch, Fisher, Tucker, Walsh & Chassman, 1993). The timing was truly fortuitous. I was asked to become a member of the first advisory committee to the first director of Recipient Affairs hired in the NYSOMH, and within the next year I was chosen to become her counterpart in the most populous region defined by the state office, New York City.

Just five years before, I could barely find evidence of the C/S/X movement and barely any formal literature on the subject of their cause. By 1994, there were dialogues and papers about the value of these once buried views, and the number of states that had created offices of consumer affairs had grown to nearly 30. On a personal level, a dream I hadn't dared imagine had been actualized: I held a position of significant stature in a major mental health bureaucracy for which my psychiatric history was the main requirement.

Was this not good news? Isn't having someone on the "inside" just what we've needed all these years? What was wrong? Why did

I feel odd, outnumbered, and worse, tolerated, especially when I refused to be a link, but insisted on being a door that opened NY-SOMH to many more people with psychiatric labels. A friend who is a sociologist reminded me that I was at the table only because it suited the current needs of those in power, and that as soon as that need was fulfilled, I could just as quickly be disinvited. How that comment dampened my hopes for being a partner, no less influential, and yet wanting and needing to believe we could transform the system from within, I realized more fully the necessity of strong outside alternatives.

My education on the job taught me about the kind of tokenism I'd only heard of from friends and former colleagues who were members of other cultural minority groups. I learned that being heard did not mean anything about being effective, particularly when the bottom lines of all decisions were control of money and the *appearance* of giving people what they need. I learned that whatever theory is in vogue is given a structure and a name, and that's what gets funded this year, no matter what else has or hasn't worked in the past, and that those who can apply the greatest political pressure will likely get the contract. Sound cynical?

Well, this year "consumers" are IN; what shall we do when they're OUT? Be honest: wouldn't some of you be relieved? Relieved to be able to do your job as you were taught and keep a place in a hierarchy that's comfortable? Perhaps not, but I suggest that the phenomenon of "involving the consumer" is already devolving, and without addressing why, we'll be part of keeping institutions alive and designed for staff control. For while my thesis confirmed that the C/S/X movement fits the definition of a self-help/mutual support network, it also unquestionably identified a civil rights movement–some refer to it as the last. Simultaneously with budgets cut so drastically that people can think of little else but to fight them, the rights of people labeled with mental illness are being systematically curbed, very soon after the few they have were won. In New York state, the out-patient commitment pilot project, a law in many states already, with open, routine exchange of clinical and criminal records, are examples of what no amount of money can change: that people believed to be mentally ill do not have the same rights to choice, privacy, or knowledge of when their sentence will end.

A piece could be wholly devoted to these excruciating facts of life for those labeled; but I hope the danger of the times will be just clear enough for you to fight with and for those you've opted to work with, rather than to let their rights either revert to zero or be "beside the point" of your work. I hope you can more fully realize where you stand, and whether how you interact with clients and co-workers perpetuates or helps to heal the pain of their status.

What I suggest is basic: facing one's fears, our healthy and less useful defenses, to check for any displaced boundaries that cause us to be other than empathic and respectful. See if you agree that the only real way for the system to become humane is for us to strive within it for the most open, compassionate, and clear relationships–with clients, colleagues, and ourselves. This means asking whether we'd rather lose a limb than control of our thoughts, and giving an answer that includes what we really feel when we meet one who has lost contact with our reality. It means looking for the commonalities among us rather than the differences that we discern by diagnosis. It means never trying to simplify what can only be holistically viewed as intricate and complex. It means never assuming, and always hoping.

What follows is another stream along these lines that I was honored to write as Class Poet in 1990 at Smith College School for Social Work. It is full of that campus' imagery where I was lucky (and indebted) enough to study in the summer semesters of what I called "Ivory Tower Social Work." It might help to know about the pond (literally called Paradise) in the middle of campus–a beautiful sight to walk around and meditate near–that was dredged the year of my class's commencement. It also might help to know that Smith is heavily psychodynamic in its orientation–but that's not why the trees are labeled all over campus. It's also a botanical garden center where the trees, flowers and birds transport one daily out of self-centered concentration into views of sky meeting treetops. It was so hard to know what to say; I hadn't written any poetry (or been so raw) for several years, but here's what emerged. I thank you for the chance to speak with you here in what is obviously a monologue, but which may lead to some dialogue wherever you are. Perhaps if we always begin with dialogue in its truest sense we'll always have the chance to end with poetry.

LETTER FROM THE EDGE OF THE STREAM

Let me speak now while I'm lucid
Like a living will, I wish you to take these words to heart.
Remember while I ramble that recognition is the beginning,
That without this we would all remain perpetually longing,
Gibberish our only language.

It is no garden of roses
Nor is it only of thorns–this I know.
Help me to see when I ought to refuse
Entry into the maze of hedges which,
Before they were clipped into order,
Were heavy with blossom,
And the scent of a season that yields
Enough heat so we rise in its waves
Heady with purpose, able to say
I did not build this wall around the open meadow.

But knowing the heartache of its entrapment is
Also of my making, and my father's,
I will join in dismantling its every brick,
Untangling its rusted wires in the rain
Of sorrow we have caused each other.

Do not be afraid to face me, letting in
  the color of my struggling skin
  the past diagnoses, the lost love for my like kind,
  the violence I drink to keep under
  that has now become the hallmark
  of my stance in the world.
My children who are dirty, my house under a tree,
  on a bench, the marks on the inside of my arm
  the scars from earlier treatments marking my brain.

If you are afraid to walk with me
My night terrors will find their way into day.
If you will not look with me, my dreams
Will remain indistinguishable by day.

At some indiscernible point, I will accept
That paradise and its demise was delusion.
But do not pretend that we are kind
To those still caught up in waking
From the dream of equal endowment.
Thus when I return lucid again
Having adopted your faith,
But day after day feels meaningless
Yet I remain fearful of the demanding more (than macrame,
Than medication), do not condescend to my slow way to readiness.

Remember I was told to strive in the same way
For the numbing of the demon's lures, by adjusting,
That I knew better than to acknowledge them
Who got the better of me and forgot that
Once acknowledged it is a long way back.

If you let me know somehow
That you willingly dredge your own pond
Of what will not erode of its own accord,
That you, too, look at the layers of silt,
The ingrown mosses near the island
Where the heron once landed,
Chose to free the choking fishes that gasped
As the surface, which was one with the depth,
Risen into mounds so dense and numerous
The boats could no longer navigate to the falls,
And let go the last look at paradise yourself,
  I'll believe you.

Let me say then while I'm loose
Like a contract broken, I wish all these words
  were unnecessary.
And remember if I begin to sound lucid again
It will be because you recognized me:
Not out of book but in a mirror
That reflected the genesis of all our longing,
The passages of our perpetual thirst to be
Nursed with cool water and a steady hand

Appearing in the confusion of hedges all uneven,
Ponds reduced to rivulets and muddy,
Walls unwillingly beaten against until broken,
Passion gone awry and held in check,
Work that never fulfilled but healed,
Language that never sufficed,
Heartache, deep sleep, and awakening again.

This is no garden of roses
But flowers thriving with thorns
with you near.

REFERENCES

Auslander, M. W. (1990). *Voices from the ex-patient movement: Psychiatric survivors unite and heal.* Unpublished master's thesis, Smith College School for Social Work, Northhampton.

Blanch, A., Fisher, D. Tucker, W., Walsh, D., & Chassman, J. (1993). Consumer-practitioners and psychiatrists share insights about recovery and coping. *Disability Studies Quarterly, 13* (2), 17-20.

When Do I Disclose?
ADA Protection and Your Job

David Schneider

SUMMARY. The Americans with Disabilities Act of 1990 (ADA) heralded a new era of civil rights for the disabled, including the mentally ill. This article concerns Title I of the ADA, protections against discrimination in employment. It is a revised version of an article orginally published in a consumer publication, the *MDSG/New York Newsletter* (Mood Disorder Support Group) to provide guidance on the pro's and con's of making disclosure of mental illness in the job environment. As such it is a valuable reference for both therapists and service recipients who wish to learn more about how the ADA relates to the employment of people with mental illness and who may be faced with the difficult decision of whether or not they

David Schneider is former Co-Director of the Consumer Information Network in New York City, was newsletter editor and board member of the Mood Disorders Support Group/NY (1994-1997), and continues as a group facilitator. A member of the NYC Task Force on Medicaid Managed Care, he has worked on consumer response systems in Medicaid managed care for the Urban Justice Center's Mental Health Project. Mr. Schneider also serves on the boards of the Picnic for Parity, an annual event in New York's Central Park advocating full parity for mental illness in health and disability insurance; and Pathways To Housing, an innovative housing provider for homeless persons diagnosed with mental illness.

Address correspondence to: David Schneider, 570 Fifth Street, #3, Brooklyn, NY 11215-3588 (E-mail: herblisa@ultinet.net).

Note: This article will not reflect any release of new EEOC guidance, court decisions, and other events that may have occurred since the article was accepted for publication (September 1997). Please consult resources on ADA Title I for the most current information.

[Haworth co-indexing entry note]: "When Do I Disclose? ADA Protection and Your Job." Schneider, David. Co-published simultaneously in *Occupational Therapy in Mental Health* (The Haworth Press, Inc.) Vol. 14, No. 1/2, 1998, pp. 77-87; and: *New Frontiers in Psychosocial Occupational Therapy* (ed: Anne Hiller Scott) The Haworth Press, Inc., 1998, pp. 77-87. Single or multiple copies of this article are available for a fee from The Haworth Document Delivery Service [1-800-342-9678, 9:00 a.m. - 5:00 p.m. (EST). E-mail address: getinfo@haworthpressinc.com].

77

should disclose their condition and request reasonable accommodation. Occupational therapists should be well-informed on this topic, to assist consumers with questions on disclosure, reasonable accommodations and other aspects of Title I. Employers can benefit by providing them with information about appropriate accommodations. And occupational therapists can advise both consumers and employers on how a psychiatric illness may affect work performance. *[Article copies available for a fee from The Haworth Document Delivery Service: 1-800-342-9678. E-mail address: getinfo@haworthpressinc.com]*

WHEN DO I DISCLOSE?
ADA PROTECTION AND YOUR JOB

In December of 1995, I organized a panel discussion presented by the Mood Disorders Support Group/NY, entitled, "Getting a Job, and Keeping It." Inevitably, employment protections under the Americans with Disabilities Act of 1990 (ADA) came up for discussion. The three panel members and many in attendance were aware that the law entitles one to "reasonable accommodation" at work. Then someone asked, "If I want a reasonable accommodation at my job–whenever I need one–when do I have to tell my boss I have a disability?" A real-life question. There were differences of opinion and uncertainty about the answer, and no one could speak from experience.

Many believed disclosure of a disability must come when beginning a new job, whether or not you're asking for an accommodation at that time. That was not my understanding, but I could not say so with certainty. It seemed to me that some of this uncertainty was due to confusion in making distinctions between what would be the *safest* time to disclose to protect against inadvertently invalidating one's rights (i.e., when one *should* disclose), what would be the *most advantageous* time to disclose, and when one *must* disclose. Since I was determined to learn what the law said, I volunteered to find as definitive an answer as possible.

The Americans with Disabilities Act is in many ways the civil rights act for the disabled. The aspect of the law discussed here, known as Title I, prohibits discrimination in all aspects of employment against individuals with almost all disabilities. If some type of "reasonable accommodation" can enable you to do your work under circumstances in which your disability is creating significant difficulties, you no longer have to hear, "I'm sorry. We tried to give you some time to straighten out, but it's not working out. I have no choice." Not only is discrimination prohibited, but your employer is *obligated* by this law to consider a reasonable accommodation geared to the specific needs created by your disability, which will enable you to perform the tasks necessary to do your job. This is truly an amazing step forward. For all who suffer from a psychiatric disorder and know how difficult it can be to function at work when trying to cope with symptoms, Title I offers a sensible and strong tool that will help many to remain employed. It is your responsibility, however, to know enough about the law to benefit from its protections should such a situation arise in your own employment.

WHEN TO DISCLOSE

I have since learned the law itself does not completely answer this question, but there is enough information to considerably clarify the picture. Under Title I of the ADA, employment discrimination is prohibited in all of the following areas: hiring, firing, job duties, training, promotions, compensation, benefits, vacation, sick and other leave. The most substantial arm is the requirement that employers make "reasonable accommodations." According to *Mental Health Consumers in the Workplace* (1991), a publication of the Bazelon Center for Mental Health Law, an accommodation can be loosely defined as "any change in a particular workplace environment, or in the way things are usually done, that makes it possible for a person with a disability to do the job." It is important to note that the accommodation must address the specific disability-related problem. *Depending on the job*, a reasonable accommodation might be to allow you to start your workday at 10 AM instead of 9 AM, or to give you more flexibility in using vacation days for time off. Doing some of your work at home might be another possibility. To be considered "reasonable," the accommodation must not cause the employer "undue hardship" (extreme expense, great difficulty, etc.).

Where does disclosure fit in? John Gresham, Senior Litigation Counsel for New York Lawyers for the Public Interest, points out, "It should be obvious, but it isn't always, that when you want an accommodation, you've got to disclose. The employer can't read your mind" (personal communication, December, 1995).

Under the law, your employer must know of your disability before being obligated to work on making an accommodation. Many physical disabilities are readily noted by the employer at the outset, and so disclosure is much less of an issue, as are efforts to avoid stigma. Psychiatric disabilities, however, are usually "hidden." It is only natural to want to avoid stigma and prejudice by keeping one's disorder a private matter. Says Gresham, "Taking into account the issue of stigma, for a person with a psychiatric disability that is not obvious to others, deciding when to disclose can be a complex, tactical decision" (personal communication, December, 1995).

In a chapter entitled "The BIG Question: Should I Disclose?" in his book, *Successful Job Search Strategies for the Disabled: Understanding the ADA*, Attorney Jeffrey G. Allen examines, albeit briefly, some of the options. "If you have an invisible disability that will not affect any essential functions of your job and will not require an immediate accommodation you need not–and probably should not–say anything" (Allen, 1994, p. 90).

One option he considers is simply waiting for a period of time after you've begun a new job. "This strategy gives you an opportunity to prove yourself on the job. You can feel more confident about disclosing your disability once you have earned the support and recognition of your supervisor and coworkers. The disadvantage of waiting until this time is that you may not be able to do the job well until the necessary accommodations have been made. Your disability may have already impacted your performance" (Allen, 1994, p. 89-90).

In a call to the Job Accommodation Network (JAN is one of several organizations providing toll-free phone lines for information on the ADA), Carol Means stated, "It is not necessary to disclose, unless you need an accommodation due to performance problems" (personal communication, December, 1995). At the ADA Information Line, Richard O. explained, "The person needs to decide what impact the disability has on their work. If they feel the job will create stress or anxiety, then after they're hired, they may want to speak with their supervisor. Keeping the emphasis on the fact that you can do the job is important" (personal communication, December, 1995).

D. J. Hendricks, Assistant Projects Manager, also at JAN, adds that, "You may be able to obtain a small accommodation–such as a schedule change–without specifying a reason that would include disclosing your disability. If that doesn't work, then you could make a more formal request for an accommodation" (personal communication, December, 1995). You can choose to keep your illness private as long as you don't require any accommodations. If you begin having symptoms, you can still choose not to disclose. This becomes more difficult and worrisome if the symptoms begin to adversely affect your performance. At that point, if you want to protect your right to an accommodation, you should seriously consider disclosing. Another should, this one is closer to a must, because the situation is approaching the point of no return.

The point of no return occurs when disclosure has been held off for too long. If you are dismissed from your job for poor performance, and you haven't yet disclosed, you are no longer protected. According to Wayne Outten, Esq., of the National Employment Lawyers Association, "If an employer, not knowing the reason for poor performance, decides to fire you, it is too late. You can't wait until you are dismissed and then claim your employer should have asked if you had a disability" (personal communication, December, 1995).

IF YOU DECIDE TO DISCLOSE

If you do decide to disclose, here's some advice. Carol Means suggests, ". . . if you do choose to disclose, which would typically be to your supervisor, it would be a good idea to also disclose to another person in the organization. This will offer you some protection in the case where a supervisor may claim never to have been told, or if your boss is dismissed. If you disclose verbally to your supervisor, you may wish to follow this up with a clearly written letter stating the same" (personal communication, December, 1995).

In an article in the Managers Journal column in the *Wall Street Journal* (1996), the guest columnist David K. Fram addresses the employers' side of this situation. Mr. Fram was an ADA policy attorney at the Equal Employment Opportunity Commission (EEOC) until 1996, and is the author of *The Complete Guide to*

Resolving Complex ADA Workplace Questions (NELI, 1996). He raises several questions employers may have about the ADA, including whether an employer can demand that an employee *prove* his/her right to an accommodation. His answer, with one proviso, is "Yes." Fram (1996) writes,

> Courts and the EEOC have made clear that unless the disability is obvious, the employer is entitled to medical documentation, including information about the employee's functional limitations, so that he can determine how to accommodate them. If the employee fails to cooperate with the employer's reasonable requests for information, the employee may be out of luck under the ADA. Thus, managers should carefully document their discussions with employees. Evidence of the employer's good faith or the employee's failure to cooperate can be critical in defending against an ADA lawsuit.

So, not only do we have the employee's right to request consideration of a "reasonable accommodation," we now have–in non-obvious disabilities–the employer's entitlement to a "reasonable request" for information.

Regardless of the hidden nature of many psychiatric disabilities, when asking for reasonable accommodation, "It's important to think about what accommodation you want and why," stresses Mr. Outten. He also cautions, "Remember, an accommodation is not a guarantee" (personal communication, December, 1995). If you still can not perform the basic job functions even with accommodation, you are in a precarious situation.

CASE HISTORIES OF EMPLOYERS IN PRACTICE: THE RIGHT WAY AND THE WRONG WAY

1. Before ADA: An Extremely Reasonable Accommodation

Fred Levine, an attorney who lives and works in Manhattan, has lived with bipolar disorder (manic-depressive illness) for many years. He has also been very active in a local chapter of the National Depressive and Manic Depressive Association. He is currently counsel to the executive director at Fountain House, a psychosocial clubhouse, rehabilitation and residential service organization serving individuals with mental illness. He specializes in managed care and mental health law, and policy issues, and is a member of the New York City Bar Association's Committee on Legal Problems of the Mentally Ill.

In 1984, after going through a debilitating episode of his illness, Fred was extremely fortunate in having an employer that (1) truly appreciated his value as an employee, and (2) a full six years before the ADA was signed into law, collaborated with him in devising what we now refer to as a reasonable accommodation.

Fred recalls (personal communication, September, 1997):

> In 1984, I was a member of the Continental Insurance Legal Division. Having joined the Division in 1978, I had a solid track record of accomplishments.
>
> My employer had no idea I suffered from bipolar illness. However, in December of that year, I suffered an episode of mania, followed by a depression that kept me at home for more than seven weeks. My family and I decided to tell my employer exactly what had happened.

Fred and his family were very concerned with what his employer's reaction to his illness would be, not to mention the time taken off on disability.

> Fortunately, they could not have been more supportive. I will always remember my supervisor's first comment to me: "As far as I'm concerned, there is no difference between what you've experienced and a broken leg. If you broke your leg and needed a ride home each night, we'd provide it. We will provide you with whatever you need, too."

Working together with his supervisor, a new arrangement was developed. For the first six months, Fred's job was restructured to reduce his caseload; he worked a reduced schedule; and took an extended midday break. On a case-by-case basis, some projects were referred to others, or he would obtain needed assistance from colleagues. There were also frequent meetings to monitor his workload. Once he resumed his former work schedule Fred was encouraged to take personal time whenever it was needed. "I was very fortunate. As a result, following this episode, I was able to resume my legal career. Without this assistance, I might well have joined the ranks of thousands of people with disabilities who, following successful careers, are dismissed when some form of reasonable accommodation could have made the difference."

2. Employee with Mental Disability Awarded over One Million Dollars from Law Firm Employer

In 1995, the Equal Employment Opportunity Commission (the federal agency responsible for handling official complaints of ADA violations) announced that due to staffing limits, the waiting time for preliminary investigation of the large number of complaints received was becoming exceedingly long, and the workload unmanageable (Wolinski, 1995). As a result, they were going to begin sending backlogged complaints to arbitration for resolution, and also recommend this course for new complaints. Although perhaps for other reasons, the following case did go to arbitration. It is instructive and precedent-setting.

Due to both the magnitude of the award, and the instance of a mental disability, this has been termed a landmark case. The plaintiff, who suffered from major depression, worked as an attorney in a corporate legal department employing over 30 lawyers. The arbitrator ruled that the plaintiff's request of his employer to limit his total work time to 90 hours in any two week period constituted a reasonable accommodation that should have been given a fair try.

The arbitrator awarded $1,126,000, including damages to the plaintiff, and fees and costs to the plaintiff's attorneys. The amount awarded for damages was based on "pecuniary losses and emotional pain and suffering, inconvenience, mental anguish, loss of enjoyment of life, and other nonpecuniary losses" (Wolinski, 1995). Both parties had also agreed beforehand that the arbitration decision–including any award–would have "the force of law" and be "both binding and non-appealable." (Note that Title I of the ADA has a limit on damages. This case, however, was found to violate the California

Civil Code as well as the ADA, and the California anti-discrimination statute provided for a damage award without limitation.)

CONCLUSION

In summary, upon taking a job, you have a choice regarding disclosure. You can choose not to disclose at the outset; however, keep in mind that if at any time in the future you decide to request an accommodation, you will then need to disclose. If you do begin having symptoms, or any disability-related problem, and are either concerned that this may affect your job performance, or will endure or even worsen, it may be wise to disclose. Again it is not a must, but a strong should. You can choose to continue keeping your disability a private matter even as your performance begins and continues to be adversely affected. However, if it begins to impact on accomplishing the essential functions of your job, you are in dangerous territory. Remember that if you do disclose, and subsequently refuse to comply with your employer's request for medical documentation that substantiates your disability, you may well be risking the loss of ADA protection. The bottom line and the only must is that if you haven't disclosed, and your disability has impacted your job performance to the point of dismissal, you are without grounds to claim that you should have received any accommodation.

Since making a decision on disclosure obviously requires reasoning and judgment, should these faculties be affected by your illness, you will be at a distinct disadvantage. Therefore advance preparation may serve you well in this situation. Discuss this issue thoroughly with a trusted friend, relative or therapist so they will be able to help advise you at such a point, and also seriously consider putting in writing a specific contingency plan and giving them a copy. If you do reach a point when a decision must be made, and realize you are not up to it, and reliable affordable advice is unavailable, disclosing may be the safest thing to do.

ADA RESOURCES

ADA USA Information Line	800-232-4955 (especially for non-English-speaking, booklets, list of organizations)

Job Accomodations Network (JAN) (the President's Committee on Employment of People with Disabilities) (800-342-5526)	800-526-7234 or 800-ADA-WORK (workplace accomodation, ADA questions) Computer Bulletin Board: 800-DIAL-JAN http://janweb.icdi.wvu.edu
NYS Office of Advocate for Persons with Disabilities	800-949-4232 (ADA technical assistance, literature) Computer Bulletin Board: 800-943-2323 http://www.state.ny.us/ disabledadvocate/ada.htm info@oapwd.state.ny.us
US Equal Employment Opportunity Commission (EEOC) NY District	800-669-4000 (questions, complaints, filing a charge) 800-669-3362 (publication ordering office)

Note: These agencies and organizations are not–and should not–be viewed as sources for obtaining formal legal counsel about your rights or responsibilities under the ADA. For referral to a qualified employment attorney for consultation on a specific situation: NELARS (National Employment Lawyers Association Referral Service) 212-302-0718.

ACKNOWLEDGMENTS

Prior to modification, this piece originally appeared in the January 1996 issue of the *MDSG/NY Newsletter*. The section "Case Histories of Employers In Practice . . ." was added expressly for this publication. The material "Before ADA: An Extremely Reasonable Accommodation" appeared–also prior to modification–as a longer piece written by Fred Levine in the April 1996 edition of the *Morningside-Westside Bulletin*. The author extends his thanks to Mr. Levine for permitting its inclusion here in its present form.

REFERENCES

Allen, J. G. (1994). *Successful job search strategies for the disabled: Understanding the ADA*. New York: John Wiley & Sons.
Fram, D. K. (September 16, 1996). What employers should know about the ADA. *Wall Street Journal*, p. 16.

Fram, D. K. (1996). *The complete guide to resolving complex ADA workplace questions.* NELI.

Mental health consumers in the workplace. (1991). Washington, D.C.: Bazelon Center for Mental Health Law.

Wolinsky, S. (September 1995). Law Firm to Pay Over One Million Dollars to Employee with Mental Disability. *Americans With Disabilities Newsletter,* [Americans with Disabilities] Law Desk. World-Wide Web: http://www.lcp.comlwhats new/9509010I. html#lwo, September, 1996.

Bridging the Gap:
Integration of Consumer Needs
into a Psychiatric Rehabilitation Program

Joan Feder, MA, OTR, CRC

SUMMARY. Traditional mental health practice has been challenged with the task of empowering consumers with greater control over their course of treatment. A review of one community based rehabilitation program is presented in which principles of empowerment have been integrated into the service. Current issues affecting occupational therapists are examined. *[Article copies available for a fee from The Haworth Document Delivery Service: 1-800-342-9678. E-mail address: getinfo@haworthpressinc.com]*

INTO A PSYCHIATRIC REHABILITATION PROGRAM

Empowerment of mental health consumers has developed rapidly in the last decade in response to budget cuts, reduced services, and societal emphasis on personal rights and freedom of choice. Nationally and locally there is evidence of an ever increasing number of consumer-run organizations such as the National Alliance for the Mentally Ill (NAMI), the National Mental Health Association and multiple self-help support groups. The recipients of services and

---

Joan Feder is Coordinator, Intensive Psychiatric Rehabilitation Services, New York Hospital-Cornell Medical Center, 425 East 61st Street-7th floor, New York, NY 10021.

[Haworth co-indexing entry note]: "Bridging the Gap: Integration of Consumer Needs into a Psychiatric Rehabilitation Program." Feder, Joan. Co-published simultaneously in *Occupational Therapy in Mental Health* (The Haworth Press, Inc.) Vol. 14, No. 1/2, 1998, pp. 89-95; and: *New Frontiers in Psychosocial Occupational Therapy* (ed: Anne Hiller Scott) The Haworth Press, Inc., 1998, pp. 89-95. Single or multiple copies of this article are available for a fee from The Haworth Document Delivery Service [1-800-342-9678, 9:00 a.m. - 5:00 p.m. (EST). E-mail address: getinfo@haworthpressinc.com].

their families are joining local and national groups in an effort to participate in the transformation of mental health care. On federal, state, and local levels, governments are funding new projects run by and for consumers. In addition, consumers and their families are being asked to participate in political decision making and policy development. Finally, rights of patients in licensed programs are being closely regulated by the New York State Office of Mental Health (OMH) with the belief that patients have the right to an individualized plan with full explanation of services provided (Office of Mental Health, 1993). In New York State, additional shifts in treatment are evident, such as the licensing of Intensive Psychiatric Rehabilitation Treatment (IPRT) programs designed to provide a rehabilitation option with emphasis on achieving community living goals and to provide a consumer-driven approach to treatment (Sheets, 1995).

Empowerment, Rappaport (1987) explains, is not only an individual psychological construct, it is also organizational, political, sociological, economic, and spiritual. There is, built into the term, the quality of the relationship between a person and his/her community (Rappaport, 1987). As consumer advocate, Harp (1994) wrote that empowerment means power–power to control one's own life and the conditions that affect that life. Empowerment has challenged traditional mental health practice and its control by professionals. Consumers are being encouraged to have a greater say in their treatment, and the relationship between consumer and professional has been altered.

As occupational therapists, mastery of one's environment and fulfillment of meaningful roles have always been the focus of our services. There is a significant shift, however, in our traditional therapeutic relationships as health care providers requiring us to redefine our boundaries. As Haiman (1995) commented, now we ourselves are taking on roles and relationships in new settings, which require exploration of our own adaptability within the professional arena. During the last decade, treatment has shifted away from the medical model, with occupational therapists working in the community, adapting and responding to the pressures that influence the focus and quality of mental health services. Occupational therapists have an opportunity to join and enhance the consumer movement by developing client-centered services where consumers can assume control over their lives and establish meaningful roles. Forging alliances among practitioners and consumers is crucial to our professional survival.

Responding to recent opportunities in New York State, Payne Whitney Clinic, New York Hospital-Cornell Medical Center, developed an IPRT program with the expressed goal of providing services to the severe and persistently mentally ill who need and want rehabilitation services in order to become more successfully engaged or reengaged in community living. The program is an active goal-focused rehabilitation process where opportunity is provided to develop the skills and environmental resources needed to enhance occupational, educational, living, and/or social roles. Its ultimate mission is to increase and sustain success and satisfaction with the least amount of ongoing professional intervention (Sheets, 1995). The initial development of IPRT programs in New York State was influenced by the psychiatric rehabilitation field based on a consumer-driven approach. Anthony, Cohen and Farkas (1990) describe psychiatric rehabilitation as a technology for helping mentally ill persons develop the skills and environmental supports to become more successful and satisfied in their living, learning, and working environments. One of the major shifts in programming was responding to the empowerment model and maximizing the clients'/consumers' involvement in treatment. This involved redefining our roles as professionals and continuing to work in a hospital-based program.

APPLYING PRINCIPLES OF EMPOWERMENT

The empowerment model of recovery is based on principles that have emerged from the experiences of consumers in recovery and in the independent living movement (Zinman, Harp & Budd, 1987; Deegan, 1992). Fisher (1994) and Harp (1994) have identified levels and principles of empowerment to guide in the recovery process. In response to increased interest on the state level in consumer advocacy and basic principles of empowerment, the following programmatic changes were implemented at the Payne Whitney Clinic, New York Hospital, IPRT program which serves clients on an outpatient basis from two to eighteen months at a time.

Maximizing Consumer Involvement in All Aspects of Treatment

From the outset, prospective applicants and their families are provided with information about the services available. The program's consumer brochure was developed with the assistance of current participants and an attempt was made to keep the language clear with limited professional terminology. In addition, to assist with a well-informed decision, all applicants participate in an intake interview and review course descriptions and consumer-written newsletters. Furthermore, an opportunity is provided to interview current participants and observe a day in the program. Acceptance into the program is a collaborative decision among the applicant, primary therapist and rehabilitation specialist with an agreement based on a one month trial basis.

The program emphasizes an active role for the client in treatment and in the development of self-defined goals. By providing a highly goal-directed program, clients are encouraged to identify, define, and document their own personal goals, and they are given the tools to research their options and develop a plan to attain change in their chosen environment.

FACILITATING RECOVERY THROUGH INSPIRATION OF HOPE AND CHOICE

Embedded in the program is the belief that positive change is both possible and attainable. Recovery is viewed as a continuous process with clients being able to take an active role in their own care and treatment. This is enhanced by providing meaningful choices and active participation in the selection process. Flexibility of services and adequate resources provide the clients with a sense of control and a feeling that their judgment is valued to the greatest extent possible. Critical choices are further enhanced by teaching the clients how to investigate their interests and assess their capabilities prior to entering a chosen environment.

A strong belief of the program founders is that our clients have the capacity to make an informed choice and take control of their life decisions. As therapists we provide the necessary tools to assist the client in making educated choices. Treatment is viewed as a collaborative effort where treatment plans are written jointly and the how and where of intervention are determined collaboratively. The identified time framework for achieving objectives is established on an individual basis. In addition, progress notes are written on alternate weeks by the clients, providing an opportunity for self-evaluation of progress toward chosen goals. Hope and peer support are also provided by a Speakers' Bureau and community involvement. Active consumers in the local community are invited to share their recovery stories and serve as resources for further community activism. In addition, directors of volunteer programs, housing coordinators, counselors from job development programs, and professionals are invited to share their personal stories and provide a rich array of resources to assist with planning and developing personal objectives.

Participation in Planning, Evaluation, and Decision-Making Structure of the Program

Participants are involved on all levels of the program starting with weekly business meetings where an agenda is developed with identification of issues that need to be reviewed. The meetings were established to provide an ongoing dialogue for both the clients and the treatment provider. Satisfaction ratings of the program are provided every three months including individual course ratings. Based on the ratings and feedback, programmatic changes have been made, including development of a consumer-run newsletter group and a buddy system for all new participants. Ultimately there is a high level of expectation that participants play an active role in their treatment and take responsibility for their recovery.

Participation in Civic Issues on Community, State and Federal Level

Empowerment should occur on all levels to enhance freedom of speech and to protect human rights. Because of budget cuts, threats to insurance coverage, and diminished mental health services, consumers need to become more active in civic issues. The program has provided this opportunity by involvement in local consumer-run demonstrations and letter writing to local, state, and national politicians. In addition, clients have been involved in developing community projects including voter registration drives in the mental health community.

DILEMMAS OF SERVICE

Overall, participants have indicated a high level of satisfaction with the program. A few issues, however, have arisen which are worth reviewing. A shift in perspective is required for both the individual client and professional alike in this model. Based on the philosophy of empowerment, the program challenges consumers to actively formulate goals and choose treatment options. Transitioning from a dependent patient to an independent, responsible client requires a high level of motivation and desire for change. The program attempts to stimulate new roles and to encourage a greater degree of independence. At the same time, the demands of the program, such as investigating choices, may be perceived as overwhelming and contradictory to the patient role the clients have developed over the years. Although the program assists the client in developing self-directed coping skills, the ability to adjust to this change in method requires a high level of symptom stability and rehabilitation readiness.

Furthermore, environmental choices in the community are often limited, with a paucity of available resources in job development and supportive education. Advocacy for the client has become crucial, requiring employers to take steps to overcome attitudinal barriers and acceptance of the Americans with Disabilities Act (ADA).

In this model, staff has had to reexamine basic values and assumptions regarding treatment approaches. Some have had to overcome their own personal biases and reevaluate their sense of the client. Within a medical model, the primary role of treatment has always been to improve or compensate for dysfunction. In addition, staff in a medical approach are comfortable with defined boundaries and distance because they feel protected (Haiman, 1995). Thus the shift to the broader goal of creating an empowering environment in which persons can assume control over their lives and establish meaningful roles is not easily achieved.

In addition, occupational therapists need to challenge their traditional orientation toward the mentally ill and reflect on their own style of providing treatment. Freund (1993) describes professionals with a high degree of success working with consumers in an empowering way as having a personality style with a high internal locus of control; that is, who have an attitude that managing one's life is primarily the result of internal motivating factors. Ultimately they work *with* consumers as opposed to working *for* consumers (Freund, 1993).

Incorporating principles of empowerment into a rehabilitation program does not change the essence of occupational therapy practice, but rather provides us with the opportunity to share our skills and provide a program which maximizes choices and options. As one of our clients wrote when reviewing the program, "I felt like I was in control of my life and I need that."

REFERENCES

Anthony, W. A., Cohen, M., & Farkas, M. (1990). *Psychiatric Rehabilitation.* Boston: Center for Psychiatric Rehabilitation, Boston.

Deegan, P. (1992). The independent living movement and people with psychiatric disabilities: Taking back control over our lives. *Psychosocial Rehabilitation Journal, 15* (3), 3-19.

Fisher, D. (1994). Health care reform based on an empowerment model of recovery by people with psychiatric disabilities. *Hospital and Community Psychiatry, 45*(9), 913-915.

Freund P. (1993). Professional roles in the empowerment process: "Working with" mental health consumers. *Psychosocial Rehabilitation Journal, 16* (3), 65-73.

Haiman, S. (1995). Dilemmas in professional collaboration with consumers. *Psychiatric Services, 46* (5), 443-445.

Harp, H. (1994). Empowerment of mental health consumers in vocational rehabilitation. *Psychosocial Rehabilitation Journal, 17* (3), 83-89.

New York State Office of Mental Health. (1993). Adapted amendments of 14 NYCRR Part 587. New York.

Rappaport, J. (1987). Terms of empowerment. Toward a theory of community psychology. *American Journal of Community Psychology, 15*: 121-148.

Sheets, J. (1995). New York-Medicaid financing of psychiatric rehabilitation services. *Community Support Network News, 9* (2), 5-6.

Zinman, S., Harp, H. T. & Budd, S. (1987). *Reaching across: Mental health clients helping each other.* Riverside, CA: Self-Help Committee, California Network of Mental Health Clients, 1987.

The Internet and World Wide Web as a Resource for Mental Health Occupational Therapists

Margaret C. Blodgett, MS, OTR

SUMMARY. The Information Superhighway, the buzzword referring to the Internet and World Wide Web system, is a new resource for occupational therapy. Therapists are discovering how the Internet and World Wide Web can allow them to access the information that they need for research, treatment planning, education, communication, and leisure pursuits. This article describes how the Internet and World Wide Web work, defines terms and tools common to these new technologies, and gives some specific locations that an occupational therapist may find useful. References are shared that relate to general mental health resources and occupational therapy in mental health resources. *[Article copies available for a fee from The Haworth Document Delivery Service: 1-800-342-9678. E-mail address: getinfo@haworthpressinc.com]*

"We are truly in an information society. Now more than ever, moving vast amounts of information quickly across great distances is one of our most pressing needs" (Kehoe, 1996, p. 1). Telecommunication is the process of using computers to communicate over distances via phone lines, networks, and satellites with other computers. "The productivity of an occupational therapist today de-

Margaret C. Blodgett is Instructor, Occupational Therapy Program, Concordia University Wisconsin, 12800 North Lakeshore Drive, Mequon, WI 53097 (E-mail: blodgetm@execpc.com).

[Haworth co-indexing entry note]: "The Internet and World Wide Web as a Resource for Mental Health Occupational Therapists." Blodgett, Margaret C. Co-published simultaneously in *Occupational Therapy in Mental Health* (The Haworth Press, Inc.) Vol. 14, No. 1/2, 1998, pp. 97-105; and: *New Frontiers in Psychosocial Occupational Therapy* (ed: Anne Hiller Scott) The Haworth Press, Inc., 1998, pp. 97-105. Single or multiple copies of this article are available for a fee from The Haworth Document Delivery Service [1-800-342-9678, 9:00 a.m. - 5:00 p.m. (EST). E-mail address: getinfo@haworthpressinc.com].

97

pends on the successful implementation of a variety of mass market information technologies" (Smith, 1996).

WHAT IS THE INTERNET?

The Internet is a network of computer networks which allows for communication between any of the machines on the networks. The networks link computers all over the world using modems (computer devices for telecommunications), telephone lines, and satellite links. These publicly funded networks are locally owned and operated. The system functions by cooperation between these local networks.

The concept of the Internet originated in 1969 as a system that the Department of Defense created for communication between several major computing centers ("Internet 101," 1996). The idea was that with a system of locally operated networks there would be no one, "main" computer that would be susceptible to damage from a natural disaster or armed conflict. In 1983 parts of this system were made available to the general public which marked the actual beginning of the Internet as we know it today (Reed, 1996). In 1992 the World Wide Web (WWW or Web) was created (Reed, 1996). The Web is actually another part of the Internet. If you access the Web you will interact with information that is graphically displayed and generally is more user-friendly than the text-only sites found on the Internet. The Web uses a linking process, called hyperlinks, to connect two locations. You will point and click (with a mouse or other pointing device) to text or graphics that have attached hyperlinks and you will then see a new location (called a Web Page) appear on your computer screen.

HOW DOES THE INTERNET WORK?

Anyone is welcome to access the Internet community, but they must have a computer that runs a standardized communication protocol, Transmission Control Protocol/Internet Protocol, (TCP/IP). This protocol allows different types of computers (i.e., Macintosh and IBM) to communicate with each other. When a message is sent from one computer it is broken down into smaller pieces of data called packets. The packets travel independently from one computer to another until they reach the final destination, where they are reassembled into the original message. Even if one or more phone lines or networks become unavailable, the message will reroute through different lines and networks to reach the target destination.

If you access the Internet you will be able to communicate with other computer users throughout the world by using tools such as electronic mail and real time typed conversations, known as Internet Relay Chat. You will also be able to access a wide variety of information and entertainment which may, or may not, be accurate, relevant, or useful. There are also a number of tools that will help you in your search for information. Some of those tools are described in this article; other descriptions can be found in any Internet introductory text.

WHAT EQUIPMENT DO I NEED?

In order to access the Internet you will need a computer, a piece of hardware called a modem, and one or more pieces of software. The modem may be a card that is installed inside the computer system (internal modem) or an external modem that is a separate component that is plugged into the back of the computer. This component allows for the digital signal of the computer to be translated into the analog signal of telephone lines and back again. Many new computer purchases include an internal modem as a part of the basic system package. If you are purchasing a modem you want to get the fastest one that you can afford. The speed capability of the modem directly effects the amount of time and money you will spend accessing information over telephone lines. These days the "33,600 bps" (bits per second) modem is the common speed purchased.

Telecommunication software is required to communicate with the modem and generally is included with your computer or modem purchase. This software allows for dialing the phone number and establishing the connection with the remote computer that you are contacting. Additional software may be needed depending on what connections you are making with your computer. Your Internet service provider may require a specialized piece of software which they usually will provide free of charge. Access to the Web is generally done by using a "Web browser" software program. This software may be purchased locally or "downloaded" (copied to your computer) from the Internet. The cost varies depending on what software you choose and what your purpose is for using the software. Educators, for example, may download some pieces of software free of charge, if their main purpose is to educate others.

HOW DO I ACCESS THE INTERNET AND WORLD WIDE WEB?

Once you have the correct equipment you will then need to find an Internet service provider. This is the link between your computer and the rest of the Internet. Some people have access to the Internet through work or school. Usually these people can then "call in" from their computer at home to their work computer and access the Internet from there. Others will have to connect though a commercial on-line service (such as America Online, CompuServe, Prodigy, The Microsoft Network, or a local company). These companies provide their subscribers with access to a vast amount of information that appeals to a variety of interests in addition to access to the Internet.

WHAT DOES THE INTERNET COST?

No one person or company owns the Internet so you do not have to pay to use it. However, there is an expense involved in connecting to it. If you have access through work or school, that facility established a connection to a local Internet network by installing the appropriate lines and software. If you do not have this type of access you will use a commercial on-line service and be charged a monthly fee that provides you with a certain amount of time per month to access both the service provider's information and the Internet. Once you have established a connection to the Internet there is no charge for actually using it, no matter where in the world your messages are "traveling."

WHAT CAN I DO ON THE INTERNET?

Some of the information available on the Internet includes text documents (references, short papers and some full text articles), graphics (drawings, illustrations, photos), video (film clips and full length features), sound (audio clips and music), and computer programs. The tools for interacting with this information include electronic mail (E-mail), Internet Relay Chat (IRC), Newsgroups, Listservs, File Transfer Protocol (FTP), and Telnet.

For many people E-mail is the most useful and widely used feature of the Internet (Collins, 1995). Electronic mail is a tool that provides for composing, sending, and reading typed messages. Anyone with access to the Internet has an electronic mail box on the computer of their Internet service provider. Mail can be sent to that mailbox from anywhere else on the Internet and the messages will be held until that person has the time to log-on (sign in) and read the messages. He/she can then respond to the message, forward the message to someone else, save the message for later reference, or print the message at his/her leisure. The term E-mail refers to both the process of sending and to the messages being sent ("I will E-mail you that information" or "I received your E-mail on that issue"). If you have an E-mail account you will be given an E-mail address. The address consists of two parts, the user name (usually some version of your name or nickname) and the domain name (Pitter, Amato, Callahan, Kerr & Tilton, 1995). The domain name will have several parts to it, separated by periods. Generally, the domain names include a name for the computer that holds the mailbox, a name for the institution, and the type of institution. The user name comes first, followed by the @ symbol and the domain name. For example (Pitter et al., 1995), jdoe@computer.institution.edu would be the E-mail address for Jane Doe that is stored on the system named "computer" at the facility named "institution" which is an educational facility. You need to be careful with E-mail addresses because they are often case sensitive. If you typed in JDOE for the mailbox in the example the message might not get delivered.

Similar to E-mail is Internet Relay Chat. IRC involves the same process as sending an E-mail message; you type a message and then send it through the networks to its destination. However, with this type of messaging the messages are all sent to a common program, called a client, and anyone with access to that same program can respond to the message and "chat" (send messages back and forth) with the sender and whoever else is on-line at the time. An example of IRC is the OT Forum held by subscribers to America On-Line at 8:00 p.m. (ET) on Mondays (Collins, 1995).

Newsgroups are electronic bulletin boards (computers) where information is posted about a particular subject. If this subject is of interest, you can log-on to a bulletin board system and read posted messages and/or post your own messages.

Listservs are automated systems that provide subscription services. People subscribe to a mailing list related to a particular interest and then receive E-mail messages from others who have subscribed to the same list. Subscribers can also send messages to the list.

File Transfer Protocol is a tool that allows for the transfer of files from one computer to another. If you want to copy, or download, a file from another computer you will use FTP. TELNET is a tool that allows a user to log-on to a remote computer. This tool allows for the opportunity to be on one computer system and do work on another. For example, use the telnet command to log-on to the Library of Congress computer to do a literature search.

WHAT WOULD I DO ON THE WORLD WIDE WEB?

The information available on the Web is similar in type to what is on the Internet, text documents, graphics, video, sound, and computer programs. The Web, however, allows the user to view those resources in a more graphical view and provides more "user friendly" ways to complete tasks than the tools mentioned above ("Internet 101," 1996). "The Web is fast becoming the largest source of network traffic around the world" (Kehoe, 1996, p. 77).

Once you have established contact with your Internet service provider (ISP), you will access another piece of software, called a Web browser. This software will allow for interaction with the graphical interfaces on the Web. Some examples of Web browsers include Mosaic, Netscape Navigator, Microsoft Internet Explorer, NetCruiser, WebExplorer, or one that is a part of your ISP software.

The Web consists of Web sites (locations) that have both text and graphics. These sites are called Web pages and there may be any number of Web pages on one computer. The typical set up is to have the first screen seen at a particular site be the "home page." From the home page you can then move to other Web pages by pointing and clicking with the mouse on hypertext (text with a connection to other locations). The destination may be on the same computer or on a different computer. Creating a Web page is not hard but requires some time to learn the basics of hypertext markup language (HTML), the background information that tells the computer how the page should be displayed. There are also software packages available that make the process for creating a web page even easier. Some of these include Abode's Pagemill and Microsoft's Front Page.

Another type of software, a search engine, is used to find locations of interest on the Web. This software can be purchased but is also available for no charge through your ISP or your Web browser. Some examples of search engines include Lycos, Magellan, Excite, and Yahoo. These software programs allow you to type in the terms for the information that you are looking for and then the program searches through the networks it has access to and brings back any addresses that have content that matches your search terms.

WHAT WILL I FIND ON OCCUPATIONAL THERAPY AND MENTAL HEALTH?

If you are a new user to the Web you may want to start by going to a general site to learn some of the basics of moving around on the Web. Try http://www.boutell.com/faq/ which gives you answers to the most "frequently asked questions" (faq). Do you need to do a med-line search? Try the address (http://www.medmatrix.org/SPages/Medline.stm), that advertises access to "Free Medline."

Occupational therapy is represented on the Web in a number of sites. AOTA has a web page that can be found at (http://www.aota.org). Another location you may want to access to start browsing for occupational therapy sites is http://otpt.ups.edu/ (the occupational therapy and physical therapy programs at the University of Puget Sound). This Web site contains many hypertext links to other related sites and provides access to lists of OT related Internet/Web addresses. Occupational Therapy Internet World at http://www.mother.com/~ktherapy/ot/ is a good resource for OT sites world wide and contains OTDBASE, a database of all journal article abstacts that have been published in 11 occupational therapy journals from 1970 to the

present. This database has been created by Marilyn Ernest-Con-
ibear, MA, OT(C), retired professor of occupational therapy at the
University of Western Ontario, London, Canada. This site also
gives information about a new Internet Relay Chat channel on
occupational therapy that is available daily to any interested parties.

There are several references to mental health and OT on these
pages, including the Association of Occupational Therapists in Mental Health, an association based in the United Kingdom. The Web
address is (http://www.iop.bpmf.ac.uk/home/trust/ot/aotmh.htm).

Some other resources related to mental health issues in general
include the Web page for the National Alliance for the Mentally Ill
(NAMI), (http://www.nami.org/) which includes information on
membership, books, conferences, medications, research, among other topics. The Mental Health Association's address is (http://
www.nmha.org/).

If you are interested in receiving and sending E-mail related to
the OT field and mental health issues, you may want to subscribe to
one of the following listservs: OCCUP-THER, OT-PSYCH, and
OT-PSYCH DIGEST. For specific information on how to subscribe to these lists, refer to the detailed information at (http://
www.mother.com/~ktherapy/ot/otspef.htm). Kristin Levine also has
written a column called "Internet Update," that appeared in several
issues of volume one of OT Practice magazine. These columns
cover details on what is available on the Internet/Web for OT and
tips for accessing various tools.

HOW CAN I USE THE INTERNET
AS A TREATMENT RESOURCE?

Consider using the Web as a resource for your consumers. Refer
them to sites that contain information that would be of interest to
them. If computers are available within your treatment environment, consider using Web activities as a treatment tool that can
enhance self-confidence, increase communication skills, and educate your consumers on a wide variety of topics. Teach clients
techniques for using the Web or let them teach you what they know.
Use E-mail to establish pen pals with people around the world. Use

Web resources to create a newsletter that clients could research and produce. The possibilities are only limited by your imagination!

The term "Information Superhighway" has been used to describe the Internet and just like the actual highway system, the Internet is always under construction and gets heavily traveled at certain times of the day. Be prepared for waiting, having to re-try addresses several times, and finding new resources when previous ones are shutdown or moved. Be aware that resources posted on an Internet or Web site may or may not be reliable references with valid information. Adhere to good research review techniques and validate all references and resources found.

Laura Farr Collins (1995) states in the premier issue of *OT Practice* "the very nature of the Internet means new user groups appear and disappear daily (or sooner), so to stay current you should conduct your own searches and explore fringe groups" (p. 40). Enjoy your 'Net Surfing and Web Browsing!

REFERENCES

Collins, L. F. (1995). OT Practitioners on line making the internet work for you. *OT Practice, premier issue, 1*, 40-45.

Internet 101 guide to understanding "Net Speak." (1996, October). *PC Novice, 7*, 34-37.

Kehoe, B. P. (1996). *Zen and the art of the internet.* Upper Saddle River, NJ: Prentice Hall.

Pitter, K., Amato, S., Callahan, J., Kerr, N., Tilton, E. (1995). *Every student's guide to the internet.* San Francisco: McGraw Hill.

Reed, K. L. (1996, April). *Basics of surfing the internet.* Short course presented at the annual conference of the American Occupational Therapy Association, Chicago, IL.

Smith, R. (1996). The on-ramp to the occupational therapy electronic superhighway. *AOTA self paced clinical course: Technology and occupational therapy: A link to function.* Bethesda, MD: AOTA.

Current and Future Education and Practice: Issues for Occupational Therapy Practitioners in Mental Health Settings

Deborah Walens, MHPE, OTR/L, FAOTA
Peggy Wittman, EdD, OTR/L, FAOTA
Virginia A. Dickie, PhD, OTR/L, FAOTA
Kathleen R. Kannenberg, MA, OTR/L
Jeffrey L. Tomlinson, CSW, OTR/L
Olivia Unger Raynor, PhD, OTR

SUMMARY. This article describes a national study conducted by the American Occupational Therapy Association Mental Health Spe-

Deborah Walens is Clinical Assistant Professor and Academic Fieldwork Coordinator, Department of Occupational Therapy, College of Associated Health Professions, University of Illinois at Chicago, 1919 West Taylor Street, MC811, Chicago, IL 60612.

Peggy Wittman is Associate Professor, East Carolina University, School of Allied Health Sciences, 306 Belk Building, Greenville, NC 27858.

Virginia A. Dickie is Assistant Professor and Director of Occupational Therapy, Eastern Michigan University, 328 King Hall, Ypsilanti, MI 48197.

Kathleen R. Kannenberg is in private practice in mental health, 202 West McGraw Street, Seattle, WA 98119.

Jeffrey L. Tomlinson is Community-Based Clinician, Washington Heights Community Services, 37 Woodcrest Avenue, White Plains, NY 10604.

Olivia Unger Raynor is Coordinator of Occupational Therapy, Director of National Arts and Disability Center and University Affiliated Program, University of California, Los Angeles, 300 UCLA Medical Plaza, Room 3330, Los Angeles, CA 90095-6967.

[Haworth co-indexing entry note]: "Current and Future Education and Practice: Issues for Occupational Therapy Practitioners in Mental Health Settings." Walens, Deborah et al. Co-published simultaneously in *Occupational Therapy in Mental Health* (The Haworth Press, Inc.) Vol. 14, No. 1/2, 1998, pp. 107-118; and: *New Frontiers in Psychosocial Occupational Therapy* (ed: Anne Hiller Scott) The Haworth Press, Inc., 1998, pp. 107-118. Single or multiple copies of this article are available for a fee from The Haworth Document Delivery Service [1-800-342-9678, 9:00 a.m. - 5:00 p.m. (EST). E-mail address: getinfo@haworthpressinc.com].

cial Interest Section to assess the adequacy of mental health content and fieldwork experiences in occupational therapy educational programs preparing graduates for current and future mental health practice. The results of the study indicate that occupational therapists, especially those who practice in mental health settings, must become more "business-oriented." This orientation includes educating occupational therapy students about reimbursement issues, legal and political systems, marketing strategies, and advocacy roles. Other recommendations are discussed as possible ways to prepare future practitioners more effectively for roles in community-based settings. *[Article copies available for a fee from The Haworth Document Delivery Service: 1-800-342-9678. E-mail address: getinfo@haworthpressinc.com]*

INTRODUCTION

The Mental Health Education Task Force was convened on November 13-15, 1992, in response to a need identified by the American Occupational Therapy Association (AOTA) Mental Health Special Interest Section Standing Committee to "assess mental health content and fieldwork experiences in educational programs to determine adequacy in providing the knowledge and skills necessary for current and future practice" (Walens, Dickie, Tomlinson, Raynor, Wittman, & Kannenberg, 1995, p. 7). Preliminary reviews of several historical documents were done as preparation for the study. This review included: the surveys and final report of the Occupational Therapy Commission on Education, Pediatric Core Curriculum (Henderson, 1991); reports of other AOTA task forces that dealt with mental health issues in the profession, and association reports dealing with mental health issues (Allen, 1975; Garibaldi, 1984); the October, 1991 Report of the PEW Health Professions Commission, *Practitioners for 2005* (Shugars, O'Neil & Bader, 1991); and minutes of the Mental Health Special Interest Section Standing Committee, the *Mental Health Specialty Interest Section Newsletter* from 1980-1981, and *Mental Health Special Interest Section Newsletter* from 1982-1988.

METHODOLOGY

A qualitative research methodology was used to provide information from a variety of sources to answer the Task Force's questions about knowledge and skills relevant to current occupational therapy practice in mental health, what was currently taught in occupational therapy curricula, and what knowledge and skills will be needed in future practice. The data collection method used was focus groups. Krueger (1988, p. 18) states that focus groups "create a permissive environment that nurtures different perceptions and viewpoints, without pressuring participants to vote, plan, or reach consensus." Non-directive interviews were used and assisted the researchers in identifying trends and patterns. Non-directive procedures began with limited assumptions allowing interviewees to talk freely about mental health practice while sharing their multiple realities.

Based on literature of how to do focus groups, several criteria were used in selecting respondents. Representation from occupational therapy practitioners in mental health, academicians who teach mental health and non-mental health content, and students was solicited. Both certified occupational therapy assistants and registered occupational therapists were included in the sample with geographic distribution in all regions and in 25 different states. A total of 48 clinicians, 20 academicians, and 9 students were interviewed.

Five focus groups were held one each in Richmond, Virginia; New York City, New York; Ypsilanti, Michigan; Chicago, Illinois; and Los Angeles, California, and four were held during the 1993, American Occupational Therapy Association annual conference in Seattle, Washington. Guidelines were developed for the interviews and the same series of questions were asked in each group. All focus groups were audiotaped and field notes were taken by one of the Task Force members. The tapes were then transcribed and reviewed. After a thorough review of all transcripts, the following nine major themes were identified and used to code and further analyze the data.

1. Occupational therapy's ability to move into nontraditional settings
2. Characteristics of mental health occupational therapy
3. Splits in the profession
4. Education and preparation

5. A sense of what is not being said or statements said without conviction
6. Current state of practice, encompassing the changes and evolution occurring
7. Characteristics of the future
8. Elements of practice
9. Choice of practice (Walens et al., p. 8).

Each transcript was then re-read and coded lines of all transcripts were entered into a file for analysis of frequency and distribution of the code within the nine themes. The final review and analysis resulted in the following major findings.

RESULTS

The first finding was that the parameters of mental health occupational therapy practice are still unclear. Occupational therapists are unable to define themselves, the foundations of their practice, and the expected outcomes of their services. A theme occurring throughout the groups was that occupational therapists and certified occupational therapy assistants in all areas, and perhaps especially in mental health, are unable to effectively define themselves to other professionals, administrators, insurance companies, managed care providers, and consumers. A non-mental health educator stated, ". . . not being able to educate . . . about how you best describe your skills . . . it's not real clean yet as to why we're better than the others, or how we have more of a holistic view, or how we can look at the activity in a different way" (Walens et al., p. 18). Another person said, "You have to figure out some way to market occupational therapy so it's exciting, appealing, and challenging to people" (Walens et al., p. 19). Participants expressed some confusion about the roles and functions of occupational therapy in short-term inpatient units. For example, occupational therapy is "not making a difference" because the focus is on medical stabilization. There were statements that suggest that occupational therapy practitioners remain focused on long term rehabilitation goals despite the realities of shorter lengths of stay. While there are practitioners who are excited about their practice and feel challenged to use a range of skills, at the same time many expressed concerns about the current realities of present occupational therapy practice in mental health and the need to transition to a community-based practice. Although measurable functional treatment outcomes appeared to be lacking in mental health occupational therapy, many participants expressed that occupational therapy's ability to analyze activity and focus on functional outcomes was indeed "what we do best." The concern was raised that too often occupational therapists concentrate their treatment interventions on components of functional skills and never apply these components to the actual functional performance required of the consumer. One therapist pointed out that psychiatric occupational therapy has more status within the pediatric treatment team than in the adult team because the assessment tools are so much better. The idea that tools help create a professional identity was discussed in conjunction with respondents' comments about the necessity for outcome measures which will help create a more viable and valued role and identity for mental health occupational therapy. With a touch of humor, one clinician commented that what mental health occupational therapy really needs was to fabricate a "brain splint" which would work immediately and effectively (Walens et al., p. 27). In general, the respondents expressed that for occupational therapists to survive, especially those working in mental health, they needed to know how to focus treatment on functional outcomes, how to measure change, and how to document functional changes of consumers for enhancing coverage and reimbursement.

The second finding was that mental health, as a core component of all occupational therapy and as a practice specialty was not adequately reflected in academic and fieldwork education, practice, the American Occupational Therapy Association and state association activities, printed materials, and communication efforts. In one group a participant stated, "I have friends in other OT schools where they might have just a very few mental health classes. Right from the beginning I think you get the message, mental health is not as important as phys dys. I mean not even considering the quality of the classes or the quantity or times of the classes, just the fact that less of an emphasis is placed on it, so it must not be important; and then why do I want to go into mental health?" (Walens et al., p. 12).

As one educator stated, "We need to be more fluid in terms of moving from phys dys rehab practice and psychosocial practice." Tying this finding to the broader issue of a "multi-skilled occupational therapy practitioner," another commented, "There's this physical disability that doesn't come attached to a psychosocial component . . . I don't think we view (ourselves) as multi-skilled." Some of the non-mental health educators who also function as fieldwork coordinators expressed their frustration with fieldwork facilities which were not willing to incorporate psychosocial and emotional goals into traditional rehabilitation programs. One participant emphasized that while psychosocial and emotional goals on rehab units should be the norm, "When you try to make that connection there are very few clinicians that are willing to go along with you" (Walens et al., p. 13). In one group, nonmental health educators discussed at length the detrimental effects of what they called the practice areas' "boxes" which practitioners create for themselves. These practice boxes limited a therapist's ability to treat the whole person and to function as a generalist.

The mental health educators summarized some of the discussion about splits or "boxes" between practice areas by emphasizing the importance of appreciating the psychosocial aspects of activity analysis for all clients and knowing something about brain anatomy, brain chemistry and the research that is being done in neuroscience. It was noted that physical disabilities clinicians are often required to treat persons with schizophrenia, cognitive problems, or head injuries and that effective practice requires an understanding of psychopathology. The mental health clinicians in several instances expressed their frustration with the American Occupational Therapy Association for its perceived emphasis on non-mental health practice areas was evidence by its lack of mental health coverage in brochures, recruitment materials, and continuing education programs. One group member stated, "The real problem is coming from AOTA . . . mental health practice is not given the same level of respect and acceptance as phys dys practice" (Walens et al., p. 12). The importance of emphasizing the psychosocial core of occupational therapy as essential to the profession's identity was discussed. One mental health educator felt that having a solid sense of occupational therapy's identity was fundamental to developing

competent practitioners, "Students have to have a very strong conceptual understanding of OT; what is occupation; what is function.
And it's not about *we do this particular type of thing in this type of
setting*. It's a much more integrated understanding of occupation
and function" (Walens et al., p. 16).

The third finding was that the culture of occupational therapy
education and practice has relied on a medical model of practice
and has not developed effective models of education and practice
for community-based services. When asked to describe practice in
the future, focus group members described it on a range from non-
existent to radically different. They agreed that mental health services will be primarily in the community, but questioned whether or
not occupational therapy will be included in the delivery. The need
for occupational therapy practice to expand into community mental
health care was emphasized by all participant groups. Three specific myths within occupational therapy culture were recognized as
creating barriers to the necessary behavioral changes which would
allow the occupational therapy profession to successfully move to
community mental health.

The first myth was that occupational therapy is defined and valued primarily as hands-on direct treatment. This frame of reference
creates problems as the role of higher paid professionals in community settings are not primarily direct service roles. In order to receive competitive salaries, occupational therapists in community
practice will need to function more often as consultants, educators,
and leaders. Interestingly, many practitioners did not see themselves
fulfilling these roles when asked to envision where they would be
practicing in the future. A strong theme in focus groups was that an
occupational therapy career was a long evolutionary process grounded
in extensive "hands-on direct patient care experience." One student
saw herself in five years still doing direct care because . . . "five
years from now is not that far away and I think that before I would
feel comfortable moving on . . . I want to get all the experience I can
with hands-on, with direct supervision" (Walens et al., p. 17). Other
students were quick to agree with this, and there was a pervasive
sense that consultation was not an entry-level skill. The essential
question posed by focus group members was, "How green is an
entry-level OTR?"

The model of the dependent new graduate doing direct treatment with direct clinical supervision for at least a few years was well ingrained in the value system of occupational therapy practitioners and was related to the second myth of our culture that students must be socialized by initially working in a hospital setting through a long, closely supervised, dependent process. So while participants recognized that community and home settings will dominate practice in the near future, the opportunity for students or entry-level practitioners to acquire the necessary skills to work in the community are very limited.

There was a third related belief which permeated occupational therapy culture; effective treatment is perceived as a process that changes the client's condition and takes place on an individualized basis. One clinician discussed the ethical decision she made regarding direct patient care when she realized that serving as a consultant could help so many more people. "I don't see that the community and the mental health system or the health delivery system can afford OTs in a direct service role. . . . It's an ethical decision. . . . I have a choice to treat one or two patients or do I have a choice to educate and treat four or five hundred when that's how many people are in the community. I feel it would be unethical to only do direct service" (Walens et al., p. 29).

The fourth finding was that to be recognized as a team professional in community mental health, a master's degree was essential (Walens et al., p. 22). Presently, the majority of leadership roles in community settings are filled by other professionals with a minimum of a master's degree in fields such as social work and psychology. Related to this finding was a pervasive theme found throughout the groups that occupational therapy practitioners must find ways to empower themselves to effectively make the transition into community based practice. Along with the ideas already discussed in this paper, as health care continues to move out of traditional institutional settings and into the community, focus group members see a role for occupational therapist as program leaders.

DISCUSSION

These findings raised many questions and issues about the present and future state of occupational therapy practice in mental health. As the practitioner who has elected to practice in the community because of ethical reasons has done, other clinicians will need to examine their assumptions regarding the nature of change in mental health consumers and to what extent occupational therapy facilitates this change and/or assists consumers in adapting to their environments.

If occupational therapy is to compete in an environment which values clinicians who hold master's degrees and are able to work autonomously, we must examine how we currently train students to become dependent practitioners who believe that supervision from experienced therapists is requisite to entry-level practice. We must develop strategies of change to empower new graduates to be independent and function not only in hospital environments but in the community. Professions such as engineering and teaching expect graduates to function independently and take on leadership responsibilities after a period of internship or training similar to that received by occupational therapists. Perhaps occupational therapy curricula need to examine the expected environments where new graduates will work and assure graduates that they have the knowledge and skills to successfully function in emerging practice environments. Additionally, the idea of the entry-level master's degree should be revisited and may be critical to the survival of occupational therapy practice in mental health and other areas of practice where professionals need to be competent in not only direct service but indirect service and consultation.

Learning the knowledge and skills inherent in assuming leadership roles should be incorporated into occupational therapy curricula from the beginning of the educational process. This curricula content should include not only understanding the organization of service delivery within state and national reimbursement systems and health care and mental health care systems, but entry-level practitioners need to learn how to assess, plan, and implement programs that serve the consumer needs of the system. Understanding practice paradigms, such as the psychosocial rehabilitation model on one hand and legislation processes on the other will be critical to survival. Both consumer and legislative advocacy and understanding and knowing how to influence policy decisions in your internal and external environments must be addressed in educational programs.

The results of this study indicate that if occupational therapy is to survive in the mental health care system, it must become "business oriented." Such an orientation includes the effective use of marketing skills, reimbursement strategies, and outcome measures. It is interesting that although the role of certified occupational therapy assistant was not often addressed, one respondent group spoke strongly in favor of using COTAs as effective service delivery personnel in community-based settings and emphasized that this is a cost effective way to do business in a community environment.

Additionally, if the business of occupational therapy in mental health care is to be successful, occupational therapists must become empowered. Occupational therapy practitioners must learn how to assume power and effectively use it. Academicians and clinicians must be cognizant of empowerment processes and provide opportunities for students and practitioners to appropriately assert and experience empowering relationships with each other which will in turn help therapists empower themselves with internal and external constituent groups.

CONCLUSION

In 1975, another Mental Health Task Force made the following statement after analysis of issues faced by mental health practice: "The problems identified in mental health occupational therapy pose real potential threats to the survival of occupational therapy. However, they are not overwhelming because we have the time and the ability to deal constructively with these conflicts" (Allen, 1975). Unfortunately, the problems identified in the 1995 study are not dramatically different from the concerns raised in 1975. Twenty years ago the committee felt that time was on their side and practitioners had time to respond to the practice dilemmas they faced. Today this is not the case as change is occurring at an accelerated pace. To quote Walens et al. (1995):

The issues represented in this study are extremely complex and are influenced by the professional, social, financial, and historical events and issues in occupational therapy and health care. Consequently, the resolutions are not simple and involve a pulling together of the whole profession. The authors believe that mental health is a microcosm of the broader contexts of occupational therapy practice as practice evolves into the 21st century. We feel strongly that, if the occupational therapy profession chooses not to listen to the "voices" of the practitioners, educators, and students who shared their views in this study then we may lose what historically has been the foundation of our profession. If we ignore the psychosocial aspects of what we do and are not explicit in documenting psychosocial aspects of intervention in all practice, these aspects will become obsolete artifacts of our history. Our challenge is to clearly articulate and demonstrate our uniqueness in order to be valued by professionals, providers, consumers, and each other. Mental health occupational therapy is at risk. The course of its future will be determined by the power and influence that individual therapists, educational programs, and state and national associations use to change the present course. (p. 5)

ACKNOWLEDGMENTS

The authors would like to acknowledge the AOTA Executive Board for their support in the funding of this study and Susan Haiman and Virginia Stoffel, the chairpersons of the Mental Health Special Interest Section from 1991-1994 and 1995 to the present, respectively, for their leadership in believing in the importance of the study. Also a special thank you to all the practitioners, educators, and students who willingly shared their perspectives and whose voices helped us understand the current dilemmas of mental health practice and the directions of future practice.

REFERENCES

Allen, C. (1975, July). *Issues in mental health OT practice* (Report of the Mental Health Task Force). Bethesda, MD: American Occupational Therapy Association.
Garibaldi, J. J. (1984, April 6). *Integrated action plan for occupational therapy in the field of mental health (Interim Report to the Executive Board of the American Occupational Therapy Association)*. Bethesda, MD: American Occupational Therapy Association.

Henderson, A. (1991). *Report of the Occupational Therapy Commission on Education, Core Curriculum Task Force*. Bethesda, MD: American Occupational Therapy Association.

Kreuger, R. A. (1988). *Focus groups: A practical guide for applied research*. London: Sage Publications.

Shugars, D. A., O'Neil, E. H. & Bader, J. D., (Eds.). (1991). *Healthy America: Practitioners for 2005*. Durham, NC: The Pew Health Professions Commission.

Walens, D., Dickie, V., Tomlinson, J., Raynor, O. U., Wittman, P. & Kannenberg, K. (1995). *Mental health special interest section education task force report*. Bethesda, MD: American Occupational Therapy Association.

Learning Contracts and the Use of Goal Attainment Scaling (GAS) for Occupational Therapy Students on Mental Health Fieldwork: An Integrated Approach to Fieldwork Learning

Anne Hiller Scott, PhD, OTR, FAOTA

SUMMARY. To counteract stereotyped views of the mentally ill and to empower occupational therapy students on their mental health clerkship, students developed individualized learning contracts. The contract required formulating their educational goals as a series of graded steps structured through the use of a sequential numerical scale, Goal Attainment Scaling (GAS) (Kiresuk & Sherman, 1968). Goals were related to the students' social-emotional concerns and anxieties encountered in this practice area through an affective GAS

Anne Hiller Scott is Director, Division of Occupational Therapy, School of Health Professions, Long Island University-Brooklyn Campus, 1 University Plaza, Brooklyn, NY 11201.

Dr. Scott adapted and used the GAS learning contract process for occupational therapy students on fieldwork while teaching mental health practice courses at the State University of New York, Health Science Center at Brooklyn, College of Health Related Professions, Occupational Therapy Program, Brooklyn, NY 11203.

[Haworth co-indexing entry note]: "Learning Contracts and the Use of Goal Attainment Scaling (GAS) for Occupational Therapy Students on Mental Health Fieldwork: An Integrated Approach to Fieldwork Learning." Scott, Anne Hiller. Co-published simultaneously in *Occupational Therapy in Mental Health* (The Haworth Press, Inc.) Vol. 14, No. 1/2, 1998, pp. 119-127; and: *New Frontiers in Psychosocial Occupational Therapy* (ed: Anne Hiller Scott) The Haworth Press, Inc., 1998, pp. 119-127. Single or multiple copies of this article are available for a fee from The Haworth Document Delivery Service [1-800-342-9678, 9:00 a.m. - 5:00 p.m. (EST). E-mail address: getinfo@haworthpressinc.com].

also known as a comfort scale. Task skills were addressed via a psychomotor/cognitive GAS. Students took an active role in monitoring their progress on their GAS while exploring emotional reactions. Through the use of an interactive log format, students received ongoing feedback and support from the academic instructor while honing their performance and clinical reasoning skills. Students often articulated a positive transformation of their views of the mentally ill and their sense of efficacy and comfort in working with this population fostered by success with their personal goal achievement on their GAS. *[Article copies available for a fee from The Haworth Document Delivery Service: 1-800-342-9678. E-mail address: getinfo@haworthpressinc. com]*

Academic and clinical educators alike are faced with the challenge of providing a meaningful educational experience in mental health that will not only impart the educational basics but also, address relevant attitudinal and affective issues to provide students with a more favorable view of this practice area. Ideally students will translate this clinical exposure to sensitive psychosocial interventions regardless of their ultimate specialty choice.

LITERATURE REVIEW

Students' Attitudes Toward the Mentally Ill and Specialty Choice

Several authors have dealt with the issue of the stereotypical and negative perceptions of occupational therapy students related to mental illness, and some researchers have suggested that the curriculum has minimal impact on students' attitudes (Burra, Kalin, Leichner, Waldron, Handforth, Jarrett, & Amari, B., 1982; Graessle, 1997; Lyons & Hayes, 1993; Page 1987; Scott, 1995; Wittman, Swinehart, Cahill & St. Michel, 1989). Since occupational therapy students are not exempt from pervasive societal stereotypes, these must color practice preferences.

For many students their choice of practice specialty may be made prior to admission (Wittman, Cahill, Swinehart & St. Michel, 1989) or may be formed prior to Level II Fieldwork (Scott, 1995). In a longitudinal study of 273 students, 71% made their specialty choice prior to Level II fieldwork with the majority expressing an interest in physical disabilities practice (Scott, 1995). This pattern was reversed however, for those who chose mental health, confirming the saliency of the fieldwork experience. For the 13.5% of the group who indicated a mental health specialty preference, more than half or 57% changed their original preference from physical disabilities or undecided based on exposure to the Level II fieldwork. Other research has been supportive of the positive impact of the fieldwork experience on both Level I and II on specialty choice (Christie, Joyce & Moeller, 1985; Ezersky, Havazelet, Scott & Zettler, 1989).

Students' Affective Responses to the Clinical Experience

Literature from nursing education is informative in shaping a phenomenological view of students' entry into the clinical setting (Beck, 1993; Kelly, 1993; Kleehammer, Hart & Keck, 1990; Pagana, 1988; Windsor, 1987). These studies highlight students' fears and anxiety level related to clinical exposure. Descriptive research on student nurses' first clinical exposure in many ways is consonant with the author's evaluation of occupational therapy students' entry process in psychosocial fieldwork.

In a qualitative study of nurses' responses to the initial clinical experience, Beck (1993) noted that the following themes emerged: experiencing pervasive anxiety, feeling abandoned, encountering reality shock, envisioning self as incompetent, doubting choices, and uplifting consequences. Pagana (1988) also focused on the initial clinical experiences in the medical-surgical area, which revealed themes related to the following threats: personal inadequacy, fear of making errors, fear of the clinical instructor, a feeling of being scared or frightened, and fear of failure. Kleehammer and colleagues (1990) corroborated high anxiety levels related to the first clinical experience and fear of making mistakes. Windsor (1987) proposed a sequence of stages in the professional development of nursing students. The initial focus of students was skill development with perceptions related to the newness of the setting and feeling scared. In this first stage students were uncertain of themselves and felt quite dependent on their clinical instructors. The second transitional stage involved a struggle to identify with the role of the nurses, followed by the third stage where students felt more comfortable in task performance and were able to take a broader view of their role.

One could draw parallels between these studies and those in occupational therapy which highlight a developmental process related to clinical reasoning moving from procedural or task focus to a more interactive and ultimately conditional model (Cohn, 1989; Niestadt, 1996) and to the evolution of cognitive skills (Schwartz, 1984) and supervisory relationships (Frum & Opacich, 1987).

LEARNING CONTRACTS AND GOAL ATTAINMENT SCALING

Learning contracts have long been a staple of professional education in structuring an active role for the student in the clinical setting and for professional development (Boyd, 1979; Cross, 1996; Knowles, 1986; Malkin, 1994; Martin, 1994; Mazhindu, 1990). Recently the use of Goal Attainment Scaling (GAS) has been documented for several professions for basic and continuing education (Cusick & Ottenbacher, 1994; Fleck & Fyffe, 1997; McAllister, 1996). The author has coupled learning contracts with GAS and an interactive log on the Level I mental health fieldwork (Scott, 1994). The value of an interactive log for occupational therapy students on mental health fieldwork has been documented by Tryssenaar (1995).

AN INTEGRATED APPROACH TO FIELDWORK LEARNING

To facilitate students' ability to address their learning in the affective domain and to recognize their legitimate struggles with intense anxieties and fears, coupled with their desire to be effective and to master skills, a system of using a learning contract and weekly log was developed. Students used GAS as a format to grade or sequentially structure goals for the Level I mental health clerkship (Scott, 1984). This integrated approach has given students a venue to explore emotional concerns and evaluate their psychological growth as well as their performance skills in the mental health setting, ultimately contributing to their ability to feel effective and to experience a sense of achievement.

GAS was developed by Kiresuk and Sherman (1968) as an approach to program evaluation in community mental health settings. It is a method of goal definition and measurement which has proven effective in articulating objective goal statements relevant to mental health settings, as well as to a variety of clinical and educational forums. As formulated by Kiresuk and Sherman, GAS provides a framework for establishing goals prior to treatment. To summarize the process as it was originally formulated, the therapist or screening therapist evaluates the patient. Goals can be mutually negotiated with the patient, or set independently by the therapist. Goals are identified and a graded goal scale is formulated for each goal area. Patients are randomly assigned to various groups or treatments. At a designated follow-up interval, goal scales are scored, and a determination can be made related to treatment or program effectiveness. The various goals can also be assigned weights to indicate priority. Auditing results of the scores for each scale yields a measurable score, which can be presented as a standard score representing a t value. This score is an index of outcome effectiveness. Summary scores indicate an improvement from the baseline score.

To elaborate on the scaling process, a graded scale is devised for each goal. This scale represents a sequence of five progressive steps or scale points, ranging from -2 to $+2$. It is possible however, to have only two or three scale points. Numerical values are assigned to each scaled statement progressing from: -2 = much less than expected outcome, -1 = less than expected outcome, 0 = expected outcome, $+1$ = more than expected outcome, $+2$ = much more than expected outcome. These values correspond to a normal curve, with 0 representing the mean and other values representing standard deviations from the mean. For those who are interested in the mechanics of calculating outcome scores, see the author's earlier publication (Scott & Haggerty, 1984). Ottenbacher and Cusick (1990; 1993) have elaborated on the measurement qualities and clinical applications of GAS.

To identify the focus for the GAS learning contracts, students engage in a process of self-assessment reviewing prior feedback from academic, laboratory and clinical areas and completing Niestadt's (1996) inventory on "Analysis of Therapeutic Self" (p. 682). They also reflect on their exposure to their first week in the mental health clerkship. To develop a goal for the cognitive/psychomotor area, students use the work sheet, "Setting A Goal" (Scott & Haggerty, 1984). Students also focus on their emotional response or level of comfort/discomfort in the clinical setting for the affective/comfort GAS. With another worksheet for the GAS Learning Contract, they complete the following areas:

1. *Goal*: A statement of the skill they wish to learn/refine
2. *Purpose*: Discuss why the goal is important to them
3. *Definition of Terms*: Each concept in the Goal Statement is operationally defined (in behavioral/measurable terms) for the Cognitive/Psychomotor Scale, the parameters of the Affective/Comfort Scale tend to be more subjective therefore students are not required to define these concepts in measurable terms but qualitatively or descriptively
4. *GAS*: The sequence of five graded steps ranging from -2 to $+2$ are rendered for the two areas Psychomotor/Cognitive and Affective/Comfort. It is noted that a GAS score of 0 is the desired goal, i.e., "expected outcome"
5. *Method*: Relates to what the student will be doing to work on their goal, i.e., the what and how of their learning process
6. *Progress Data*: The student records their ratings daily using the GAS and reflects on their objective/subjective experience in the weekly log.

Most students focus on goals for their GAS concerned with the therapeutic use of self and how to relate professionally to patients based on the norms of mental health practice, such as initiating conversation and overcoming fear of approaching patients, not revealing personal information, focusing conversation on patients' therapeutic goals, setting limits, providing reinforcement and feedback, leading groups assertively, and so forth.

Through the log and progress data GAS ratings the instructor provides critical feedback, support and monitors progress. There is a midterm review, and generally it works best for students to continue to solidify their progress by working on the same goals. In a summary log assignment, students review their experience and incorporate their comments related to articles by Lyons and Hayes (1993) about occupational therapy students' stereotypes of the mentally ill, by Schwartz (1984) on students' own cognitive development and by Tryssenaar (1995) focusing on the log-related learning process. The implications of this experience for future fieldwork and professional development is then summarized. Samples from students' GAS scales and log summary are illustrated in the articles in this volume by Lieberman (1998) and Raymond (1998).

The majority of students report in the summary logs the benefit they experienced from having to take a process view of their learning over time. Most develop a richer view of the mentally ill as three dimensional individuals, contrasted to earlier unidimensional stereotypes. Students develop confidence in their ability to sensitively relate to psychological content in the clinical setting. The measurable aspect of GAS is very reinforcing for supporting the student's effort in their own process of change and growth. The process of self-monitoring is known to produce reactive changes. Research indicates that: (1) reactive changes are greater if only one behavior is monitored, (2) self-recording is more effective than a third party's recording, (3) social reinforcement and feedback contingent on self-determined performance goals enhances reactivity, and (4) motivation produces a facilitatory effect in modifying behavior (Ciminero, Nelson, & Lipinski, 1977; Nelson, 1977).

The benefits of GAS are consistent with principles of adult learning in harnessing self-directed initiative. This process is not a substitute for on site supervision and the benefit of working with experienced role models. However, it does put the learner in the driver's seat and provides the mobility to achieve significant emotional and cognitive benefits in a challenging practice area.

REFERENCES

Beck, C. T. (1993). Nursing students' initial clinical experience: A phenomenological study. *International Journal of Nursing Studies, 30*(6), 489-497.
Boyd, E. M. (1979). Contract learning. *Physical Therapy, 59*(3), 278-281.
Burra, P., Kalin, P., Leichner, P., Waldron, J. J., Handforth, J., Jarrett, F. J. &

Amari, B. (1982). The ATP-30–A scale for measuring medical students' attitude toward psychiatry. *Medical Education, 16*, 31-38.

Christie, B. A., Joyce, P., & Moeller, P. (1985). Fieldwork experience, part I: Impact on practice preference. *American Journal of Occupational Therapy, 39*(10), 671-674.

Ciminero, A., Nelson, R. O. & Lipinski, D. P. (1977). Self-monitoring procedures. In Ciminero, A., Calhoun, K. S., Adams, H. E. (Eds.), *Handbook of behavioral assessment*. New York: John Wiley & Sons.

Cohn, E. S. (1989). Fieldwork education: Shaping a foundation for clinical reasoning. *American Journal of Occupational Therapy, 43*(10), 240-244.

Cross, V. (1996). Introducing learning contracts into physiotherapy clinical education. *Physiotherapy, 82*(1), 21-27.

Cusick, A. & Ottenbacher, K. (1994). Goal attainment scaling: Continuing education evaluation tool. *Journal of Continuing Education in Health Professions, 14*(3), 141-154.

Ezersky, S., Havazelet, L., Scott, A. & Zettler, C. (1989). Specialty preference in occupational therapy. *American Journal of Occupational Therapy, 43*(4), 227-233.

Fleck, E. & Fyffe, P. (1997). Changing nursing practice through continuing education. A tool for evaluation. *Journal of Continuing Education in Nursing, 18*(6), 37-41.

Frum, D. & Opacich, K. (1987). *Supervision: Development of professional competence*. Rockville, MD: American Occupational Therapy Association.

Graessle, E. A. (1997). Influences on occupational therapy students attitudes about mental illness. *Occupational Therapy in Mental Health 13*(3), 41-61.

Kelly, B. (1993). The "Real World" of hospital nursing as perceived by nursing undergraduates. *Journal of Professional Nursing, 9*(1), 27-33.

Kiresuk, T. J. & Sherman, R. E. (1968). Goal attainment scaling: A general method for evaluating comprehensive mental health programs. *Community Mental Health Journal, 4,*443-453.

Kleehammer, K., Hart, L. & Keck, J. (1990). Nursing students' perceptions of anxiety-producing situations in the clinical setting. *Journal of Nursing Education, 29*, 183-187.

Knowles, M. (1986). *Using learning contracts*. San Francisco, CA: Jossey Bass.

Lieberman, S. (1998). Inspirational beginnings in an occupational therapy mental health setting. *Occupational Therapy in Mental Health, 14*(1/2), 143-154.

Lyons, M. & Hayes, R. (1993). Student perceptions of persons with psychiatric and other disorders. *American Journal of Occupational Therapy, 47*(6), 540-548.

Malkin, K. F. (1994). A standard of professional development: The use of self and peer review: Learning contracts and reflection in clinical practice. *Journal of Nursing Management, 2*(3), 143-148.

Martin, J. (1994). Independent fieldwork: Do students value this method of learning? *11th International Congress of the World Federation of Occupational Therapists, 1*, 195-197.

Mazhindu, G. N. (1990). Contract learning reconsidered: A critical examination of implications for application in nurse education. *Journal of Advanced Nursing, 15*(1), 101-109.

McAllister, M. (1996). Learning contracts: An Australian Experience. *Nurse Education Today, 16*(13), 199-205.

Nelson, R. O. (1977). Methodological issues in assessment via self-monitoring. In Cone, J. D. Hawkins, R. P. (Eds.), *Behavioral assessment: New directions in clinical psychology.* New York: Bruner Mazel.

Niestadt, M. (1996). Teaching strategies for the development of clinical reasoning. *American Journal of Occupational Therapy, 50*(8), 676-684.

Ottenbacher, K. & Cusick, A. (1990). Goal attainment scaling as a method of clinical service evaluation. *American Journal of Occupational Therapy, 44*(6), 519-525.

Ottenbacher, K. & Cusick, A. (1993). Discriminative versus evaluative assessment: Some observations on goal attainment scaling. *American Journal of Occupational Therapy, 47*(4), 349-353.

Pagana, A. (1988). Stresses and threats reported by baccalaureate students in relation to an initial clinical experience. *Journal of Nursing Education, 27,* 418-424.

Page, M. S. (1987). Factors that influence students choice of mental health as a career. *Mental Health Special Interest Section Newsletter, 10*(3), 1-3.

Raymond, R. (1998). Fieldwork Journal at F.E.G.S. (1998). *Occupational Therapy in Mental Health, 14* (1/2), 155-165.

Schwartz, K. (1984). An approach to supervision of students on fieldwork. *American Journal of Occupational Therapy, 38*(6), 676-684.

Scott, A. (1995). *Mental health specialty preference in occupational therapy: Using the theory of work adjustment to examine the influence of values, reinforcers and job satisfaction upon the level II fieldwork affiliation.* Unpublished doctoral dissertation, New York University, New York.

Scott, A. (July 9, 1994). *Achieving goals in therapy and education.* Paper presented at the meeting of the Canadian-American Occupational Therapy Association Annual Conference, Boston, MA.

Scott, A. H. & Haggerty, E. J. (1984). Structuring goals via goal attainment scaling in occupational therapy groups in partial hospitalization settings. *Occupational Therapy in Mental Health, 4*(2): 39-58.

Tryssenaar, J. (1995). Interactive journals: An educational strategy to promote reflection. *American Journal of Occupational Therapy, 49*(7), 695-702.

Windsor, A. (1987). Nursing students' perceptions of the clinical experience. *Journal of Nurse Education, 26,* 150-154.

Wittman, P., Swinehart, S., Cahill, R. & St. Michel, G. (1989). Variables affecting specialty choice in occupational therapy. *American Journal of Occupational Therapy, 43*(9), 602-606.

Memoirs from a Mental Health Affiliation

Vladimir Sychev, OTS

SUMMARY. For students entering the Level II fieldwork experience in mental health, there is often great concern about one's ability to work effectively with the mentally ill population. Developing competency and comfort with this population is a critical area of practice and students can benefit from peer-oriented learning experiences which address their particular issues. This memoir recounts one student's log as a learning chronicle for the benefit of other students. It outlines common fears, coping skills and knowledge that are mastered during the course of practice in a typical psychiatric setting. *[Article copies available for a fee from The Haworth Document Delivery Service: 1-800-342-9678. E-mail address: getinfo@haworthpressinc.com]*

When occupational therapy students enter Level II fieldwork experience, they usually have a sufficient body of knowledge in mental health. However, students don't have stories to tell from clinical experience. These stories provide a repertoire of expecta-

Vladimir Sychev is Staff Occupational Therapist, Kingsbrook Jewish Medical Center, Occupational Therapy/Physical Therapy Department, 86 East 49th Street, Brooklyn, NY 11212.

This article is excerpted from the student journal kept by the author while enrolled as a student at City University of New York, York College, Occupational Therapy Program during his affiliation at St. Lukes-Roosevelt Hospital, St. Lukes Division, Department of Occupational Therapy, Recreational Therapy and Creative Arts Therapy in New York.

[Haworth co-indexing entry note]: "Memoirs from a Mental Health Affiliation." Sychev, Vladimir. Co-published simultaneously in *Occupational Therapy in Mental Health* (The Haworth Press, Inc.) Vol. 14, No. 1/2, 1998, pp. 129-141; and: *New Frontiers in Psychosocial Occupational Therapy* (ed: Anne Hiller Scott) The Haworth Press, Inc., 1998, pp. 129-141. Single or multiple copies of this article are available for a fee from The Haworth Document Delivery Service [1-800-342-9678, 9:00 a.m. - 5:00 p.m. (EST). E-mail address: getinfo@haworthpressinc.com].

tions and a basis for clinical reasoning that students can apply to new situations. That is why I thought that from an educational perspective this book might include some helpful hints from my clinical experience. I hope that reading these memoirs will facilitate your transition from the academic classroom environment to the clinical realities of occupational therapy practice in mental health.

It is human nature to approach new situations with a certain amount of anxiety, and entering Level II fieldwork as a student can certainly generate a tremendous amount of anxiety. Affiliating at a facility for patients with psychosocial dysfunction may prompt even greater anxiety due to the student's anticipation of working with individuals demonstrating erratic, difficult and unpredictable behavior. These preconceptions are the result of stigma attached to persons diagnosed with mental illness and occupational therapy students are no exception in having these stereotypes (Lyons and Hayes, 1993). If you are having the fieldwork experience along with other occupational therapy students, it is crucial to support each other and discuss your concerns. I felt that it was very important to give feedback to my fellow students as well as to receive it. This give and take process enhanced our productivity and effectiveness. As we learned to support each other, we became less overwhelmed while working with troubled and challenging patients.

WEEK ONE: FEAR OF THE UNKNOWN . . .

On January 6, 1997, I started my fieldwork experience at St. Luke's/Roosevelt Hospital, Department of Psychiatry. When I arrived, I realized the facility was nothing like I had envisioned. In the midst of multistory modern buildings in uptown Manhattan, the location didn't grant the kind of isolation from the general public that I had anticipated. Other preconceptions proved right. I expected to see a security guard and security indeed appeared tight.

I appeared before the doors of Clark 9 Inpatient Unit full of doubt because I felt I lacked the required finesse to work with acute mentally impaired patients. I felt uncomfortable because I didn't know what to expect nor did I know what was expected of me. Though I knew I would have to put into practice what I had learned in college about communicating with, evaluating and treating patients with psychosocial problems, I was worried about how I would deal with patients because I thought they would sense my lack of confidence in my professional performance. And, I didn't know how they would react to this discovery.

My fellow students experienced similar feelings (G. Weinstock, personal communication, January 12, 1997). Gwen wrote in her log,

> People's outlook concerning any issues is often formulated based on their first contact or initial experience with it. It takes a conscious effort to dispel preconceived notions. My initial exposure to mental illness was with a classmate who was diagnosed with manic depression. I knew her throughout a period of depression and the upward swing towards mania with psychotic features. My experiences with her were helpful in the sense that I am familiar with the symptoms of mental illness, medication and relevant patient issues. However, I also have some preconceived notions about mental illness. So I have to actively clear my mind of these notions. In addition, I cannot let my 'issues' about mental illness affect my outlook either. I realize that I should make a conscious effort to treat each patient as a 'first experience' and ensure that none of my preconceived notions affect treatment.
>
> One issue I've been having difficulty with is as follows: I like being friendly and smiling at people in general; but I am beginning to fear that it's possible that some of the patients who are curious about therapists' personal lives may misinterpret this. I realize that some patients are not entirely responsible for what they are saying; but it can be difficult to sort out what's personality and what's mental illness. So, I'm trying to work out a balance between being friendly, maintaining a healthy distance, and ensuring safety. This is a good learning experience and I will resolve it as best as I can.

Kay's (Katherine Sheehan, personal communication, January 12, 1997) log reads as follows:

> Two days into this fieldwork experience, I see my biggest challenge to be learning how to effectively communicate with low functioning patients. My concerns about my ability to be

effective here are, I believe, typical of someone new to the field who needs to learn how to work with patients in an inpatient program. At this point I have observed the patients in the hallways and in a limited number of group sessions and have witnessed a variety of behaviors. I have also had the opportunity to observe various staff members interact with patients. Most seem to use a very matter-of-fact, non-emotional approach to redirect and divert patients. I have also had the opportunity to observe three groups–two verbal and one task-oriented–which has helped me know what to expect in terms of participation and response.

I feel comfortable with my ability to plan, organize and run groups in other settings. I look forward to encountering individuals here and getting feedback on what I can do to be effective and make the best use of the short time the patients have on the unit. I do not believe that any doubts that I have about working with this population stem from fear for my personal safety, but arise rather from my lack of experience. I have a good feeling about the amount and type of supervision I will receive, so I hope to develop acceptable skills in a reasonable amount of time.

After completing one week at this fieldwork site I am beginning to know the patients and the program and to feel more comfortable in the setting. I am also beginning to understand the OT role. As I see it now our primary responsibilities are in evaluation of the patient in order to assist with discharge planning and provision of opportunities for structured interaction with others while the patients are on the unit.

I feel somewhat uneasy about my responsibilities because I do not yet have a good understanding of how the paperwork should flow. Now that I have a specific patient to follow, I will be able to see how that works. I also feel uneasy at team meetings because the people and places as well as some of the terminology is new. Some of the speakers are hard to understand. I have to concentrate very hard to follow what is being said. Chart availability can be limited because many staff members need to use the charts, and access is difficult because the nursing station is so congested. These concerns should be alleviated by continuing to work with the documentation and the patients. I also want to pursue getting information on the newer medications that are commonly prescribed.

END OF WEEK ONE:
FEELING LOST . . . AND FOUND

The experience of the first week has given me a new confidence about myself. My attitude has changed greatly since the first day. The pressure of the unknown dissipated and I felt relaxed and comfortable. Although I had only 2 patients, I felt that I didn't do enough. I felt frustrated about Mrs. K., who refused occupational therapy services and was avoiding one to one interviews and other evaluations. In addition, in her eyes I was getting worse because on Friday she saw a picture of me as her cousin's boyfriend and on Monday, I became a dope dealer and she sincerely hated me. So I have been anxious about whether or not it would be possible to establish a rapport with this patient.

I was glad that we had formal supervision on Monday, and our supervisor was able to answer questions about my patients and evaluation procedures. For example, I was clear afterwards about when I should use the various standardized occupational therapy assessments. In addition, I was relieved that my affiliation began to be more structured, because I felt a bit lost and confused about due dates for official paperwork. After the supervisory meeting, I felt more confident and I left behind all my fears. I thought that now was the time to be constructive and efficient. Yet, I still felt the need to familiarize myself with the minute details of life on the unit and in the occupational therapy department. I realized that to be competent, I had to know all the resources available for patients' treatment from therapeutic use of self to arrangement of ingredients in the kitchen cabinets in the occupational therapy department. I thought that familiarizing myself with this would be very helpful, and in the future it would allow me to determine areas of dysfunction, set goals in order of priority and implement treatment aimed to improve function.

THE WORLD ACCORDING TO THE OCCUPATIONAL THERAPY STUDENT MANUAL

During their first days at this facility students are given the Occupational Therapy Student's Orientation Manual. The purpose of this manual is to provide information regarding the type of experience offered, staff structure of the facility and its services, documentation guidelines, and the clinical expectations. The self-explanatory, structured nature of this manual may decrease the need for intensive supervision.

Remember, the process of becoming an occupational therapist involves refining a sense of professional identity (Cohn, 1989; Sabari, 1985) and using self as a therapeutic agent (Neistadt, 1996). We, as students, will bring a composite of knowledge, skills, and personal learning style to the fieldwork experience. Based on our strengths and weaknesses, specific strategies to enhance our performance will be developed. Supervision is structured to ensure high quality care for the patients while simultaneously facilitating and managing the learning process for students. Our experience at this facility will be quite challenging and the amount of information may seem overwhelming. Be prepared for the fact that working on an inpatient service can be a source of stress, misunderstanding and frustration or it can present an opportunity for students to receive an abundance of information and viewpoints, leading to a more productive work environment.

During our fieldwork experience, as an occupational therapy student, we will test first hand the theories and facts learned in academic study and refine our skills through interaction with patients and staff under close supervision in order to develop entry-level competency in areas of assessment, treatment planning, problem solving and clinical reasoning, administration, and professionalism. We would be expected to become proficient in implementing, justifying and evaluating the effectiveness of treatment plans. We will be responsible for articulating our understanding of theoretical information and identifying our abilities to implement assessment and treatment techniques. We will be demonstrating how to utilize assessment tools before we start using them. We will observe the professionals running groups before we conduct them on our own. We will be able to benefit from supervision as a source of

self-directed learning which is crucial for professional development. In our opinion, ongoing supervision provided weekly as an
essential part of the program was flexible in accordance with our
interests, needs, learning styles and abilities.

LIFE IN THE FAST LANE

Emphasis on returning patients quickly to the community requires students to maximize therapeutic efforts within limited time
frames. As a result, I have had to constantly apply time management techniques to my therapeutic endeavors with stays as brief as
10 days, as I have been required to proficiently evaluate, treat and
plan for the discharge of each patient. Most of the occupational
therapy treatment is accomplished in task-oriented and discussion-
oriented yet task-focused groups. Specific therapeutic activities
such as crafts, meal preparation, self-care groups, art, dance, music
and recreation therapy, self-awareness and assertiveness training,
work issues, leisure exploration, stress management, and physical
relaxation are offered to patients. The number of patients seen within group activities varies according to the unit population, severity
of the individual's illness and type of activities. The length of treatment sessions varies considerably, but generally are 45 minutes to 1
hour. Patients are seen in several rooms on the unit and in the
community on outings (for patients with privileges). Weekend activities are planned and conducted by patients under the supervision of
an OT/RT/Creative Art Therapy (CAT) department representative.
Special events are also offered throughout the year. Films, movies,
newspapers, and other written materials are currently offered to
patients during individual and group contacts.

Be prepared to be assigned your first patient at the end of the first
week of your fieldwork. By the end of second week, you're expected to have four patients. Each subsequent week, two more
patients will be assigned to you weekly, until you reach a caseload
of ten patients a week. It may seem scary at the beginning. However, as you progress as a professional, you will be able to handle this
caseload and paperwork. What you need to do is to take one step at
a time and remain calm and confident. Your supervisor will assist

you on your way to becoming an entry-level occupational therapist and provide the necessary supportive environment.

In addition, you will handle treatment planning with the team which includes the consulting psychiatrist, a certified social worker, registered nurses, medical residents, and psychology interns. During the first two weeks you will receive orientation from the nursing and social work departments.

In this psychiatric setting, patients' symptoms vary daily. Behavior and responses may be highly appropriate one day, yet more regressed the next day. Thus, it is important to communicate the behaviors observed by the therapist and staff for documentation. Remember, most staff have little time to read through each patient's progress notes. So, notes should be clear and concise. In addition, notes should report the patient's responses within the activities and how their behavior corresponds to the treatment goals indicated in the plan of service. It is essential, if the team members are to understand our plans, that we be clear and specific in stating our goals. Goal-setting for students and patients may sometimes be frustrating or even disappointing. Don't be discouraged if your patient doesn't reach a goal while he/she is in your care. Remember, other factors contribute to successful accomplishment of goals, including the patient's participation in the goal setting process and his/her motivation, the family, and time.

REFINING THERAPEUTIC USE OF SELF AND CLINICAL REASONING

Beside your professional growth, you need not forget why you are on site–to offer empathic care for the needs of your patients. The occupational therapy program is directed toward sustaining and protecting intact functions and abilities, improving function where possible, preventing further disability, supporting basic levels of personal growth through the use of effective collaborative evaluation and treatment. Your active vocabulary should include words like encourage, motivate, and inspire, and there also should be an element of fun. You must acknowledge patients' pain, depression, frustration, and lack of motivation. Frequently you will encounter the dilemma of unworkable or inappropriate behavior on the part of the patient. Praise, encouragement, and prompting are not always sufficient to obtain cooperation. After all, the occupational therapy student cannot force a patient to be "motivated," to cooperate with therapeutic activities and evaluations. In this case, your progress note should reflect that goals were not met or only partially met due to the patient's poor motivation and uncooperative behavior.

I was glad that as I became more experienced I was able to clinically judge the situation and determine the best action to take under various clinical circumstances. I offered consistent reward or reinforcement in the form of attention, friendly humor, outright praise, and sincere respect for positive, socially acceptable behavior and productive activity. By acknowledging patients' achievements, you will guide them toward a productive, more harmonious approach to daily life. Try to increase patients' abilities to problem solve, think before acting, and control impulses.

On the other hand, a patient who is not motivated to get well will often respond to a therapist who makes time to listen, shows genuine concern, inspires confidence and enthusiasm in the therapy process, and fully explains why the treatment is important. Remember, our clients' lives are as stressful as our own–except they are also dealing with a disability. Be ready to meet a patient for the first time and encounter an angry individual who is "held in the hospital" against his/her will. Also keep in mind, that patients with chronic mental illnesses often lose the ability to converse politely. Remember not to get defensive and offended, realizing that many factors can contribute to the anger such as fear, loss of control, and anxiety about the unknown. To diffuse the situation, let the patient express anger, listen carefully and provide reassurance that therapy will help him/her to get better and out of the hospital. Keep in mind that as therapists we learn as much from our clients as they do from us because they are a great source of knowledge and inspiration. I found it best to adopt a pleasant, soft-spoken approach in communication with patients. A louder voice will not increase understanding and will make the patient feel uncomfortable. In my opinion, some key things to keep in mind were to remain calm and somewhat formal, respectful and polite.

As occupational therapy students, we must also be aware of certain precautions while conducting therapeutic intervention. In my opinion, it is important to understand the possible side effects of psychotropic drugs and to know the medication status of each patient. Help the patient to separate his symptoms from the side effects of medication such as dizziness, exceptional drowsiness, dry mouth, and blurred vision. Explain to the patient that he or she is not getting "sicker," that side effects are usually temporary and there is medication to minimize these effects. Encourage the patient to continue to take the prescribed medication during and after hospitalization.

Sexual Harassment, Substance Abuse, and Other Taboos

Another issue which is sensitive in nature is sexual harassment because it is not an easy topic to discuss. We may or may not have had training in responding to sexual harassment. A quick review of the occupational therapy literature shows nothing formally written on this topic. There is no specific strategy for handling a patient's sexually provocative behavior. We may choose from several options in dealing with the harasser: ignore the behavior, avoid the individual, confront the patient, and always report the behavior to a supervisor and the team. One needs to consider this behavior in context with the patient's illness and treatment plan and work with the team on how to appropriately address sexual material. It is important to be familiar with the policies of the unit related to sexual issues such as the "no touching rule" which is common on many inpatient units.

Removing oneself from adverse environments and experiencing negative feelings toward a sexually harassing patient are natural reactions. The patient's sexual advances may fill you with a sense of anger, embarrassment, and humiliation. In dealing with sexually provocative behavior, you should take certain precautions with a patient who may initiate a sexual overture. One of the things you can do is ask your supervisor, a staff member or a fellow student to observe the therapy session and give feedback as to whether the patient is presenting risk. By doing this, we make others aware that we are trying to prevent sexual misconduct. We should also notify staff members of the patient's behavior. Another suggestion is to document the patient's actions in the medical chart. For instance, if the patient says something derogatory, makes suggestive or seductive statements, tries to hug or kiss you, you can protect yourself officially in the progress note. If a patient unexpectedly demonstrates sexually provocative behavior do not panic. Remain calm and try to set limits. If that does not stop the patient, calling for help is indicated.

We were asked to observe and later lead the Occupational Therapy Assessment Group designed by the occupational therapy staff of St. Luke's Detoxification Unit. This group uses a non-threatening format to explore the patients' deficits in coping skills, interpersonal skills and problem solving skills in such performance areas as workplace, family, community, and treatment facilities.

The therapist begins the group with an explanation of its purpose. Patients will have to fill out an assessment form and participate in discussion related to their feelings and thoughts about this task. The focus of the discussion is on the process of recovery and the pitfalls that await each patient in an attempt to create a lifestyle without drugs and alcohol. Herein lies the challenge. We will have to get through the denial system and guardedness, and help patients understand the realities of recovery. We want them to see what brought them here. We will give feedback to patients about how their behavior and some of the attitudes will be a liability to them as they proceed into recovery. Illusion must be overcome.

Keep in mind that each patient with a history of substance abuse is unique in their personality and interpersonal skills and that in a treatment facility without addictive substances, their real behavioral style surfaces. We will encounter patients who are not happy about being in treatment. The anger, stubbornness and rebelliousness of these patients are pervasive. We may deal with such patients by drawing attention to how their desire to criticize others without looking at their own faults is getting in the way of treatment.

Many patients with a diagnosis of alcohol or substance abuse have an intense fear of failure and/or equally intense fear of success. We should make these behaviors a topic for discussion and get other participants to give feedback to assist the patient in taking an honest look at him or herself in order to change their self-defeating attitudes. We may encounter patients who will cry during discussion. We must not ignore it. Do not panic. Try to draw the patients' attention toward the necessity to forgive and love themselves and these may be a solution to their problems. Keep in mind, we are the ones who lead the discussion. And, we will need to determine the depth of the therapeutic benefit the patients will enter into during the discussion.

TO SMOKE OR NOT TO SMOKE . . .

Another addiction problem which deserves our attention is smoking. Over the years, the solarium and corridors of St. Luke's Hospital Inpatient Psychiatric unit have been clouded with patients' cigarette smoke. However, on March 24, 1997, Clark 9 entered a smoke-free era. Smoking hours have long been part of the daily schedule on the unit, with patients demanding their next puff. And some staff probably used cigarettes as a means to keep patients calm. The main purpose for the smoking ban is to protect patients and personnel from the health risks associated with smoking and second-hand smoke. Under the new hospital policy, smoking will not be allowed on the unit. That means patients who live on locked wards will be able to smoke only when an OT/RT/CAT representative escorts them on a group walk.

The staff members realized that denying tobacco to extremely mentally ill patients can cause too much anxiety among patients, make them angry and rebellious. They recognized that smoking is an addiction. As a result, now smoking cessation programs will be a part of the treatment plan and daily activities schedule. Barring patients from smoking may seem like oppression rather than treatment. However, I believe it's time to recognize and treat nicotine dependence among individuals with mental illnesses as much as alcoholism. I think that use of tobacco will kill more of those patients who smoke, than their psychiatric problems will. Health care workers of Clark 9 came up with safer ways to administer nicotine. Though nicotine gum is a problem for psychiatric patients who chew too rapidly or who don't have teeth or dentures, a nicotine skin patch should help many quit smoking.

CONCLUSION

My fears of working with mentally ill patients diminished with continuing contact with these individuals during my affiliation. Fieldwork experience exposed me to a large array of different situations and a variety of diagnoses and/or dysfunctions as well as provided me with the opportunity to attain competence through repeated experiences. In my opinion, having an affiliation at this facility helped me develop the ability to understand how symptoms and psychopathology affect performance and functioning in the activities of patients' daily lives.

Although the learning process for me is far from over, I feel more competent in using assessment tools and evaluation procedures and more proficient in implementing treatment for psychiatric patients. As time has passed, I realized that the fieldwork affiliation on the inpatient psychiatric unit could be a rich and rewarding experience which may have a tremendous impact on a student's career choices and is an extremely beneficial educational experience. At the beginning of my internship, I didn't expect that within such a short period of time I would be able to successfully establish and sustain therapeutic relationships and to work collaboratively with others in the multidisciplinary team. The experience at St. Luke's Hospital Psychiatric Unit really benefited my education. As time passed, it frequently seemed to me that I had become so much a part of the unit team that I was hardly distinguishable from the other unit staff. By the end of my Level II fieldwork experience, I felt I had the knowledge, skills and abilities needed to be capable and ready for entry-level practice.

REFERENCES

Cohn, E. S. (1989). Shaping a foundation for clinical reasoning. *American Journal of Occupational Therapy, 43*(4), 240-244.

Lyons, M. & Hayes, R. (1993). Student perceptions of persons with psychiatric and other disorders. *American Journal of Occupational Therapy, 47*(6), 541-548.

Neistadt, M. (1996). Teaching strategies for the development of clinical reasoning. *American Journal of Occupational Therapy, 50*(8), 676-684.

Sabari, J. (1985). Professional socialization: Implications for occupational therapy education. *American Journal of Occupational Therapy, 39*(2), 96-102.

Inspirational Beginnings
in an Occupational Therapy
Mental Health Setting

Susan S. Lieberman, OTS

SUMMARY. This article includes excerpts from a fieldwork log for a student's Level I experience. The student was assigned to the Brooklyn Veteran's Administration Medical Center Inpatient and Day Hospital Program with an occupational therapist supervisor. It recounts the student's concerns, in a beginning placement, as an individual who had no previous exposure to a mentally ill population. In the course of understanding the role of occupational therapy with the benefit of a strong clinician role model, the student not only learns procedural skills in occupational therapy assessment and group leadership, but also engages in a reflective process of professional growth and begins to develop a more conditional and holistic perspective of the patients with whom she is working towards fine-tuning critical aspects of the therapeutic use of self. Through the use of a learning contract developed in the format of a Goal Attainment Scale (GAS), she formulates a goal for the psychomotor domain of improving skills in interpersonal relationships with patients focusing on using verbal and nonverbal communication for interaction in a

Susan S. Lieberman completed this journal based on the Level I Fieldwork placement at the Brooklyn Veteran's Administration Medical Center, working under the supervision of Emily Weinstein, MA, OTR/L, while a student in the Occupational Therapy Program at the State University of New York, Health Science Center at Brooklyn, Brooklyn, NY.

Address correspondence to: Susan S. Lieberman, 1189 East 9th Street, Brooklyn, NY 11230.

[Haworth co-indexing entry note]: "Inspirational Beginnings in an Occupational Therapy Mental Health Setting." Lieberman, Susan S. Co-published simultaneously in *Occupational Therapy in Mental Health* (The Haworth Press, Inc.) Vol. 14, No. 1/2, 1998, pp. 143-154; and: *New Frontiers in Psychosocial Occupational Therapy* (ed: Anne Hiller Scott) The Haworth Press, Inc., 1998, pp. 143-154. Single or multiple copies of this article are available for a fee from The Haworth Document Delivery Service [1-800-342-9678, 9:00 a.m. - 5:00 p.m. (EST). E-mail address: getinfo@haworthpressinc.com].

variety of settings. For the Affective Domain Scale (Scott, 1998), also called the Comfort Scale referring to the importance of students feeling comfortable in a psychiatric unit, the student indicates a desire to reduce her level of anxiety while working in mental health. Through the process of writing her log and weekly monitoring of the GAS goals, we follow her progress in confronting and conquering a number of challenges presented on a psychiatric unit. *[Article copies available for a fee from The Haworth Document Delivery Service: 1-800-342-9678. E-mail address: getinfo@haworthpressinc.com]*

LOG 1: ANXIETY STRIKES

On September 10, 1996 as I walked into the Brooklyn Veteran's Administration Medical Center, mixed feelings assailed me. I was really excited about the new rotation but nervous about the fact that it would be in a mental health setting. Never having worked in this setting before, I didn't know what to expect. My feelings of anxiety reached their peak as the occupational therapist turned the key, locking us in the acute psychiatry unit. Believing in introspection as a tool to better understand myself, I began to examine the numerous issues which contributed to these feelings. Initially, my mental health knowledge base is derived from prerequisite psychology classes as well as books and movies. A lot of social stigmas and preconceived misconceptions related to mental health are woven into our society's views. I am sure that I have picked up on many of these views subconsciously and, therefore, have a hard time accepting mental illness as I do physical illness.

Unintentionally, Emily, my occupational therapy supervisor, began the orientation by addressing my affective goal of feeling less anxious and more comfortable with the patients. I was paired here with another student, Eija Friedlander. Emily asked us to be participants in a relaxation group she was running and share our feelings even if they were not positive ones. I actually did participate and it really helped me realize how tension filled I was. After the session, I became a little more relaxed. This brief feeling of relaxation helped me feel slightly more comfortable in the setting.

A great deal of thought was given in considering what area I would like to grow in and choose for my Psychomotor/Cognitive Goal Attainment Scale (GAS) (Kiresuk & Sherman, 1968; Ottenbacher and Cusick, 1990; Scott & Haggerty, 1984), a part of my learning contract. This decision was made as I watched Emily administer the "Role Checklist" (Oakley, 1982) to a patient. This patient had just been admitted to the facility and the team was having a hard time getting a clear focus on the patient. It seemed that Mr. D. was a Vietnam veteran and for the past two months had barricaded himself in his apartment, not allowing anyone in. At the team meeting, Emily suggested administering the test and met with a very positive response. During the interview, interpersonal skills were the key to extrapolating important information regarding the patient's past history and present and future view of roles. I noted that part of her success was also related to the comfort level that she exhibited while being with the patient. She seemed as relaxed with him as she did with us and other colleagues she met in the hall. Mr. D. seemed to sense that relaxed and comfortable tone and shared with her his thoughts and dreams.

After observing and participating in the routine of two days in a mental health setting, the first area I would like to work on is improving my interpersonal skills. These skills are essential in dealing with the mental health population. Another focus of mine for the Affective/Comfort GAS will be to focus on lowering my anxiety level and beginning to feel more comfortable in this setting. Hopefully, these tools will help give me a better understanding of the patient, thereby, enabling me to help the patient by formulating the best and most appropriate treatment goals. The following is my GAS Learning Contract (Scott & Haggerty, 1984).

GAS (GOAL ATTAINMENT SCALING) LEARNING CONTRACT (Scott & Haggerty, 1984)

GOAL: To improve my interpersonal relationship skills and feel comfortable working with patients in a mental health setting.

PURPOSE: Good interpersonal skills will help improve my communication with the patients. This will facilitate a better understanding of my patient's profile, giving me information which I can then use to create an accurate and appropriate treatment plan.

DEFINITION OF TERMS: (Define each term used in the goals in behavioral terms if possible.)

Interpersonal Relationship Skills: Using verbal and nonverbal communication for interaction with patients in a variety of settings
Comfortable: Not feeling anxious
Mental Health Setting: Veteran's Administration acute psychiatric unit and the Day Hospital

PSYCHOMOTOR/COGNITIVE OUTCOMES–GOAL ATTAINMENT SCALE (Scott, 1998) (NOTE: Scale is on a normal curve from -2 to $+2$, reaching a score of "0" is considered normal.)

-2 Will have no communication with patients other than saying hello upon being introduced

-1 Will have communication with two patients, conversing only about niceties (the weather)

 0 Will have closer communication with at least two patients discussing any topic that may arise, while assisting the OTR who is leading the group

+1 Will communicate with one patient on a close one to one basis by administering an evaluation

+2 Will have much communication with all patients in a group while acting as a leader/co-leader

AFFECTIVE/COMFORT OUTCOMES–GOAL ATTAINMENT SCALE (Scott, 1998)

-2 Maximal Anxiety–Feeling extremely uncomfortable in mental health setting. Having a dry throat and a hard time swallowing

-1 Moderate Anxiety–Feeling reasonably uncomfortable in the setting. Having a slight dry throat and needing a drink every once in a while

 0 Minimal Anxiety–Slightly uncomfortable but beginning to relax when working under supervision

+1 No Anxiety–Does not feel anxious when dealing with a patient under my own jurisdiction

+2 Feel Comfortable–Feel relaxed and able to communicate with all patients while running a group

METHOD: I will learn through both observation (watching my supervisor) and active experimentation how to improve my interpersonal skills as well as my comfort level. I will chart my progress in my log, both successes and failures while doing evaluations, groups and general unit visits. It will be interesting to observe the grading process over time.

PROGRESS DATA: Ratings of weekly performance

The progress data ratings for this first log were Psychomotor GAS: 9/10 −2 and 9/17 −1, Affective GAS: 9/10 −2 and 9/17 −1.

LOG 2: "THE RABBI" AND THE HEALING POWER OF A CULTURALLY RELEVANT ACTIVITY

The day began with an aura of excitement. Emily said that today we would do a cooking group related to the upcoming Jewish New Year holidays of Rosh Hashanah and Yom Kippur. She explained that at different times of the year, activities would address different cultural holidays and if it was not a patient's specific cultural holiday, it was a great experience to learn about other cultures.

As we dragged all the bags of ingredients up to the Acute Inpatient Unit, Emily explained that we would be making matzo balls and matzo ball soup. She said that she had done this activity before, and it's always a big hit. We put down our bags in the dayroom where all the patients were milling around, and Emily announced our plans. Responses were very mixed. Some people were enthusiastic, while some just went back to doing whatever they were doing. One patient we called "The Rabbi" did perk up. The Rabbi had been a Jewish chaplain in the army and now was in the hospital for deep depression. It seemed that after the Rabbi retired from the army, he opened a kosher hotel in a distant vacation area. He knew how to cook and loved it! Emily knew this and asked the Rabbi to please come over and take charge of the pot in which the soup would be made. The Rabbi instantaneously assumed the role of assistant. What an interesting and sudden role reversal, from patient to assistant chef!

I had to become very task oriented, as I helped Emily set everyone up in a comfortable circle and prepared the ingredients for the patients to begin working. As cooking in general, and matzo balls in particular, is a task I am familiar with, I felt my feelings of anxiety slip away, and I began to interrelate with the patients, discussing common ground related to food and cooking experiences. This was becoming a very positive experience for me, as it was the first time in this clinical experience that I was able to move up to a +1 on my GAS for affective/comfort outcomes, not feeling anxious at all; and I was at a GAS of 0 for my interpersonal goal. Interestingly enough, the patients who had not come to participate in the activity before, were now slowly getting involved. It seemed that this pervasive positive atmosphere was drawing everyone into the group. Note-worthy, was the fact that everyone was enjoying the activity and I would assume that the anxiety levels of many of the patients were reduced during this activity, too.

The highlight of the day came when the soup and matzo balls were ready to be served. The Rabbi, who, with our encouragement and approval, had now assumed the role of leader, began to give out bowls with soup and a matzo ball to each patient and staff member alike. The joy and pride he displayed were just a sight to behold! It really warmed my heart. Everyone enjoyed the fruits of their labor, seeming to feel that they had truly completed a purposeful activity. I left the hospital that day on an emotional high! I was trying to take one day at a time, for this day I felt I had climbed my GAS, closer to reaching my ultimate goals.

I entered Emily's office the following week greeted with the wonderful news that the Rabbi had been discharged from the hospital. At the team meeting, Emily's contribution was acknowledged. It seemed due, at least in part, to the role that the Rabbi had assumed in the cooking activity. His sense of self and purpose had started to return, his depression began to lift and his road to recovery had begun. Everyone on the team seemed to have a soft spot for the Rabbi. He had had previous admissions due to depression, but as he began to feel better each time, he often helped other patients through difficult times and had the respect of patients and staff alike. News of his discharge brought a feeling of cheer into this team meeting room, a room that is often filled with the gloom of illness and suffering.

During the team meeting, Emily questioned the staff as to whether there was a patient who needed cognitive testing, as her students needed to do a cognitive evaluation, the Allen's Cognitive Level (ACL) (Allen, Earhart & Blue, 1992). Wanting us to do both the Leather Lacing Task and an activity from the Allen Diagnostic

Manual (ADM) (Earhart, Allen & Blue, 1993) to support the findings, Emily left it up to us to divide the testing sessions.

It was easy to be the analyst watching Eija administer the ACL Leather Lacing Task, but administering the ADM Recessed Box Activity Test was my challenge for the day. My hands were a bit shaky as I arranged the materials needed for the activity. I quietly gave myself encouragement saying, "Susan, you're doing great." Reading the instructions helped me stay focused and I began to relax. The rest of the testing session progressed very smoothly. A helpful tool I am learning to use to reduce my anxiety, especially when taking partial or full charge of a group or testing session for the first time, is to focus on the activity and after relaxing a bit, I can competently continue leading the session.

After the session was completed, we checked the patient's chart, collecting all the information we needed for our assignment. At that point, the day had come to an end.

LOG 3: THINGS ARE NOT ALWAYS WHAT THEY SEEM

As I walked into Emily's office, she looked up and said, "Brace yourself as I am about to tell you an unbelievable story." She proceeded to say how the FBI had come yesterday to arrest Mr. D., the supposed Vietnam veteran she had administered the Role Checklist to during my first week (Log #1). He was wanted in a few states for fraudulent check writing. They had wanted to first discharge Mr. D. and then have the FBI arrest him to spare the unit the turmoil, but the FBI came when no official staff were on duty, and the whole plan backfired. Feelings of shock assailed me.

As I entered the Acute Inpatient Unit after hearing the morning news, my anxiety levels were up once again. Feelings of doubt were also crowding my thoughts. After some introspection regarding why I was so upset, I realized that I had sat in on quite a few team meetings where there was much discussion relating to patient psychological analyses, and here a phony just slipped into the system. I finally decided that this is what experience is all about. I have a lot to learn and I need to realize that no system in the world is perfect. A consoling thought was that in the end, the system did catch up with him. I began to feel better.

Upon entering the team meeting room, Emily quietly whispered to Eija and myself that she would like us to present to the team our ACL results as well as the patient's response to last week's testing. As the team represented a room of seasoned professionals, Eija and I automatically looked at each other, reading each others eyes, sharing feelings of anxiety. Eija and I have often said how nice it is to work together, giving each other support and sharing how each felt the other performed and could improve. We understand each others goals for the learning contract and try to guide one another in attaining higher levels of success.

Apprehensively, I began the presentation, but began to relax as other team members supported our test results with findings of their own. Remarkably, some of the concerns I had were concerns the team members shared as well. One issue I raised got three comments from different members who shared the same concerns. This was a shot in the arm and a very positive experience for me.

The Day Hospital Program is another psychiatric facility at the V.A. Hospital. Emily had introduced us to the members of the group in previous weeks in the hope of us taking over the craft group in the program, which had been run by an occupational therapist who had left the facility and never been replaced. Her hopes were that we would run the group for the last few weeks of our stay. Eija and I had come up with an idea for the craft group, following the group protocol required for class. The director of the Day Hospital, a social worker by profession, had asked us to present our idea at the community meeting, as he was excited with our new input into the program.

With a great big sign and a pile of flyers, we walked in to the community meeting already in session. Only a few faces out of the thirty people sitting in the room (twenty-five members of the program and five staff) were familiar ones. Previous class presentations of the group protocol helped in giving me the confidence I needed to proceed. It was a good experience to present our project idea in front of all these people, and I feel that the more experience I have, the less nervous I'll be in the future. The response to our presentation was very positive, and later in the day, the guys (as the patients call themselves) we met asked us again when the project would begin.

My learning encounters for the day also included doing part of the readings for the relaxation group. Once again, I began with a dry throat, but as I continued to read and concentrate on the soothing words, I felt myself relax. Emily is continuing to groom us for taking over the relaxation group. She would like us eventually to run it as co-leaders. At this point Eija and I are doing all the readings for the group, and Emily is helping us with the introductory and closure segments of the meetings. The role of co-leader that I am slowly beginning to assume is starting to feel more comfortable. Still working on perfecting the pace and tone of the reading, I feel that the more comfortable I am with the skill, the less anxious I'll be.

In closing, I feel that I am fortunate to have the opportunity at this time to work on my goals which are so important for both personal and professional growth.

LOG 4: MORE OT EVALUATIONS AND LEADING OUR FIRST GROUP

In the morning, we stopped into the Community Meeting at the Day Hospital Program as the director had suggested, to remind everyone about our special "Fess Up with Painting Group" in the afternoon. The response was positive and Eija and I left feeling excited and nervous.

We cut our lunch break in half and rushed to set up the room for the group. Eija and I have similar natures which I feel works to our benefit, as we both like to be organized and prepared ahead of time. I was really excited and nervous, as this was to be my first experience in independently co-leading a group. I began the introductions with a definite pit in my stomach, following the outline I had prepared describing the activity and the group's goals. The group was attentive and the attitude seemed very positive. This helped me relax somewhat, and by the time the activity was underway, I was communicating with all the members of the group with no anxiety. The session went very well, and by the time we were finished, the group was talking about their plans for next week, as this activity is planned for three, once a week sessions. Eija and I were exhausted, but really happy that all had gone well.

Emily felt it was an opportune time to meet with the patient to whom we had administered the ACL Testing, to give him a summary of our feelings. We had discussed what each of us would ask and say to clarify certain points, and bring the testing full circle. Emily, Eija, the patient, and I sat down to talk in a quiet room. I interpreted his sentences to have sexual undertones. He had been convicted several years ago on a sexual assault charge and was even being monitored by a parole officer. He stated that he now felt ready to enter society. The whole meeting, though, left me emotionally drained, with many serious points to ponder. I shared this with Emily, and she said she was emotionally drained too. Reality hit! Even as an experienced therapist, feeling emotionally drained, and having serious concerns, was normal.

Emily had a lovely gift for us this morning. She had a pin made up for each of us, just like the one she wears, with our names on it and the department name. It's funny sometimes, that as old as we may be, putting on a name pin still had a terrific, professional feel to it.

Our group today was up to session two of three sessions in our painting series. Eija was going to do the introductions and I the closure. It really went extremely well. I was moving up on my psychomotor and affective scale, as I communicated with all the patients in a very comfortable and relaxed manner (interpersonal GAS +2 and comfort GAS +1). At this point, the group members knew my name, and I know most of theirs. This helped in having a closer connection and Emily told us from day one to try to remember as many names as you can. It really makes a difference.

The highlight of my day was definitely the administering of the Barth Time Construction (BTC) (Barth, 1988) done on the Dual Diagnosis Unit, which I had never been on before. Emily did not want me to work with only one person, but with a large group. I felt this was really a good way to measure how I was doing on my GAS scales, and I was right. It tested my GAS comfort and communication levels, and I really think I did fine. I felt much more confident than ever before, speaking to the participants in a very relaxed tone, as the testing proceeded.

Emily was really happy on completion of the test. She felt I had done very well and wanted me to administer an adaptation of the BTC the following week for those patients who were attending the

group for a second time. Her objective was to have the same participants fill out their Time Chart, displaying what would be their ideal
week post-discharge and then compare it to the original. Emily's
request seemed to mirror her pleasure and show support, which
encouraged me to keep climbing up that Goal Attainment Scale.

LOG 5: REACHING NEW HEIGHTS

As we entered the immaculately clean Acute Inpatient Unit, we
knew something was afoot. Emily informed us that there would be
an inspection on the unit today, as the hospital is looking into where
to make budget cuts. Emily's Relaxation Group was pushed up to
9:30 A.M. instead of 11:00 A.M., the thought being that the patients
would be in a group when the inspectors arrived.

Emily requested that Eija and I run the Relaxation Group, and
unbelievably I didn't even get nervous. It was just fine. Eija and I
split the readings, and Eija did the introduction and I did the closing. Emily began to comment on what group members were sharing
as I was leading them through the closing. There may have been
times in the past when I might have been a little disturbed by her
frequent interruptions, but at this point in my clinical rotation, I was
able to understand that the group discussion had taken an unusually
serious direction, and I appreciated the depth and understanding of
her comments.

The third of our three session groups of painting at the Day
Hospital was the biggest success of all! I don't remember the group
ever having such a good attendance since I began working in this
program. The air was charged with excitement and hustle bustle as
we prepared to decorate T-shirts. I felt very comfortable with this
group during both the introduction and the entire activity. I know
almost everyone by name, and they know my name too. The group
had a very relaxed and pleasant atmosphere, very conducive to
working toward achieving goals. The group ended on a very positive note, with group members sharing that Eija and I deserved a lot
of credit, as we had worked very hard and did some beautiful things
with them that they would never have done on their own.

The patient I had concentrated my attention on during the Barth
Time Construction testing last week was ready with some encour-

agement to do the second BTC suggested by Emily. When he completed the test, the patient and I moved to another table away from the group, and had a long discussion. Emily felt this would be helpful to the patient in gaining insight into what his life had been in the past, and what he would like it to be like in the future. She felt a one on one was a good idea, and after that, the patient should come and share his thoughts at the group's conclusion.

During the discussion, I really felt very calm and in control, and the whole process seemed to flow very smoothly. Looking back on my GAS where I defined Interpersonal/Relationship Skills that I would like to work on, I wrote using verbal and non-verbal communication for interaction in a variety of settings with patients. When I saw this, I felt everything come together. That was exactly what I used to communicate with this patient. My verbal skills were used to discuss the BTC Chart and have an overall discussion with him, and my non-verbal skills related to such things as my facial expressions, as I listened to the patient's life history and related problems. It was great for that moment to be on the top level of my Goal Attainment Scale, a level that I had originally questioned if I would ever reach.

REFERENCES

Allen, C., Earhart, C. & Blue, T. (1992). *Occupational therapy treatment goals for the physically and cognitively disabled.* Rockville, MD: American Occupational Therapy Association.

Barth, T. (1988). The Barth time construction. In B. Hemphill (Ed.), *Mental health assessment in occupational therapy* (pp. 115-129). Thorofare, NJ: Slack.

Earhart, C., Allen, C. & Blue, T. (1993). *Allen diagnostic module.* Colchester, CT: S&S Worldwide.

Kiresuk, T. & Sherman, R. (1968). Goal attainment scaling: A general method of evaluating comprehensive mental health programs. *Community Mental Health Journal 4*, 443-453.

Oakley, F. (1982). The model of human occupation in psychiatry. Unpublished master's research project, Virginia Commonwealth University, VA.

Ottenbacher, K. J. & Cusick, A. (1990). Goal attainment scaling as a method of clinical service evaluation. *American Journal of Occupational Therapy, 44*(6), 676-684.

Scott, A. & Haggerty, E. (1984). Structuring goals via goal attainment scaling in occupational therapy groups in a partial hospitalization setting. *Occupational Therapy in Mental Health, 4*(2): 39-58.

Fieldwork Journal at F.E.G.S.

Rami Raymond, OTS

SUMMARY. The challenge of working with the mentally ill population on the first Level I fieldwork exposure is often experienced in a setting where the on-site supervisor is a therapist from another discipline. Many skilled mental health professionals can offer a rich learning experience and assist students in mastering generic clinical skills in relating to and understanding the psychiatric population. Occupational therapy students bring to this clinical relationship the opportunity to demonstrate the effectiveness of occupational therapy interventions through group work, and individual evaluation and treatment, which benefits both the clients and the larger program. This article recounts the journal of a Level I student's journey through a setting that provided a receptive environment for fostering growth in the process of becoming truly comfortable and effective in the skills and roles of an occupational therapist in a mental health environment. *[Article copies available for a fee from The Haworth Document Delivery Service: 1-800-342-9678. E-mail address: getinfo@haworthpressinc.com]*

WEEK 1: ALL MY CHILDREN

Any trepidation I may have had regarding the mental health clerkship was quickly dissipated during my first two days at the

---

Rami Raymond completed this journal based on the Level I Fieldwork placement at F.E.G.S. (Federation Employment and Guidance Service) in Manhattan, while a student in the Occupational Therapy Program of the State University of New York, Health Science Center at Brooklyn, Brooklyn, NY.

Address correspondence to: Rami Raymond, 565 Crown Street, Apt. # 4A, Brooklyn, NY 11213.

[Haworth co-indexing entry note]: "Fieldwork Journal at F.E.G.S." Raymond, Rami. Co-published simultaneously in *Occupational Therapy in Mental Health* (The Haworth Press, Inc.) Vol. 14, No. 1/2, 1998, pp. 155-165; and: *New Frontiers in Psychosocial Occupational Therapy* (ed: Anne Hiller Scott) The Haworth Press, Inc., 1998, pp. 155-165. Single or multiple copies of this article are available for a fee from The Haworth Document Delivery Service [1-800-342-9678, 9:00 a.m. - 5:00 p.m. (EST). E-mail address: getinfo@haworthpressinc.com].

F.E.G.S. (Federation Employment and Guidance Service) continuing day treatment center.

We were met by a warm, caring and concerned supervisor, Anita Newman, who described her feelings towards her clients "as if they are my children," and assured us we were too. She understood that our lack of experience with the mental health population might engender anxieties, and her description of her clients in sympathetic and humane terms allayed a great deal of them. During the two team meetings which we attended, we were introduced (once to a round of hand clapping) and made to feel extremely welcome. I was very impressed at the intensity of concern with which clients were discussed and the feeling of trust which the staff of about twenty (mainly social workers and a few therapists, no occupational therapists) accorded their director.

Clients at the facility, mainly those with chronic schizophrenia, some with dual diagnoses, are treated with great respect and there is a philosophy, which I heard plainly verbalized, of utmost commitment on the part of the professionals serving them. Many of the clients themselves were welcoming and friendly, and by the second day were greeting me by name. They truly appreciated our presence there, and despite some obvious expressive difficulties and negative symptoms of schizophrenia, seemed eager to reach out to us and make us feel welcome. If I have dwelt on the atmosphere and associated impressions, it is because I feel that it is special and optimal therapeutically for the clients and for me as a student.

GROUPS, GROUPS AND MORE GROUPS . . . AND CONFIDENCE BEGETS CONFIDENCE!

Groups! There were thirty-four on Wednesday, each one different. We observed six and will run one next week. I am ill at ease addressing groups, therefore my focus for self development on my learning contract will center on being a facilitative group leader. I observed that the best sessions were ones where clients themselves rather than the therapist made therapeutic suggestions to one another, gave advice and voiced constructive criticism, but that happened in a structured way, with the leader guiding the group to a point they wanted it to get to, and then eliciting involvement from participants. Other therapists, who tended more to lecture than to ask for comments, ended up in verbal conflicts with the clients. I observed that a skilled leader got *everyone* involved. My goal for the learning contract using the Goal Attainment Scale (GAS) (Kiresuk and Sherman, 1968; Ottenbacher & Cusick, 1990; Scott and Haggerty, 1984) is to get more than half of the clients actively involved in the group activity and process. That will take a lot of confidence but although I may have had little before, F.E.G.S. is a place and our supervisor a person who inspires confidence, and I look forward to running a group. The learning contract that I have developed follows:

GAS – GOAL ATTAINMENT SCALE LEARNING CONTRACT (Scott & Haggerty, 1984, p. 89)

GOAL: To be a facilitative group leader as evidenced by involving most of the group members in a session.

PURPOSE: I am ill at ease addressing groups, and involving most people in a group will be evidence that I have progressed in overcoming that (because it is easy to address only the willing participants).

DEFINITION OF TERMS: (Define each term used in the goal in behavioral concepts if possible.)
Group: Collection of individuals meeting to interact and achieve a common goal.
Group Leader: Person who guides the dynamics of, sets the agenda of and dictates the tone (atmosphere) of the group interaction.
Facilitative Group Leader: Group leader, whose message is brought out by being evoked by the participants. Rather than lay down rules, he elicits their involvement on a topic or task.
Theory: That patient involvement and opinion has more influence ultimately.

PSYCHOMOTOR/COGNITIVE OUTCOMES–GOAL ATTAINMENT SCALE (Scott, 1998) (Note: Scale is on a normal curve from -2 to $+2$, reaching a score of "0" is considered normal.)
-2 Involve only participants that volunteer to join in
-1 Involve less than half
  0 Involve most participants
+1 Involve 3/4 of participants
+2 Involve all participants

AFFECTIVE/COMFORT OUTCOMES–GOAL ATTAINMENT SCALE (Scott, 1998) (Note: Scale is on a normal curve from − 2 to + 2, reaching a score of "0" is considered normal.)

− 2 Too intimidated to elicit participation of anyone except those that volunteer them

− 1 Too intimidated to elicit participation of anyone except the mildly withdrawn

  0 Confident enough to involve most participants

+1 Confident enough to involve almost all participants

+2 Confident enough to involve all participants

METHOD: Start by asking people's names and writing the names in a circle on a sheet of paper in the same place order as they are sitting. Thus withdrawn members can be called by name. I note the number of participants and put a check near their names when they speak. This gives me visual data about who has yet to speak and I know where to put my effort and I also have a way to determine if my goals are met.

PROGRESS DATA: Weekly recording of ratings for the two/three groups that I lead/co-lead.

WEEKS 2 AND 3: LEARNING BY DOING

Team meetings are a central feature at F.E.G.S. and are held twice a week for the entire staff of about 20 and on other days for subgroups of staff. Therapists take turns discussing in depth a client from their caseload for clinical and educational purposes, and the psychiatrist offers insight into various behaviors and conditions. There is frequent mention of F.E.G.S. being a "community." One manifestation of that idea was a meeting of the entire "engagement and treatment track," of about a hundred clients and staff, where clients were encouraged to step up and voice their opinions on how things should be run, their likes and dislikes, etc. I feel that this is indicative of the high degree of regard clients' interests are given at F.E.G.S.

My supervisor gave me a group to run, and two other therapists asked me to lead and co-lead groups which I agreed to do. I led a group called creative writing, whereby clients wrote on a theme I gave them for twenty minutes and then read out their work if they wished to do so. Of ten clients present, eight read out their ideas on an ideal vacation. It surprised me that people I thought were almost non-verbal in fact could express sophisticated thoughts, and that others seemed to have the language skills of children. Schizophrenia is a condition where the lack of communication due to negative symptoms can lead to deceptive appearances. That group I was happy with, and I felt it lent expression to my learning style of diverger in that I was able to generate ideas to the group about what to write, and use reflective observation in deciding when and how to encourage a client to read out their work.

In contrast, a group I led in week 3 the same day was an extremely difficult one to get clients to participate in. That was partly due to there being 28 clients and it being after lunch, but I think also because it was only a "talking" group for the "engagement" clients. I did not meet my goal of getting most clients to participate–but I feel that if the group is restructured with an activity included–even perhaps just to comment on a picture they are given–that it may help focus clients and motivate them. I suppose I anticipate using the Model of Human Occupation (MOHO) frame of reference (Kielhofner, 1992) whereby people's innate capacity for interests is used to inspire participation.

My other two groups, held in weeks 2 and 3 are crafts groups, where I interact with people when they need help or encouragement with a project. Sometimes I initiate communication with a client if they are unmotivated to engage in doing anything. It is a parallel group so interaction between members is limited, but I try to draw their attention to each others work and acknowledge it is consistent with my GAS learning contract to involve most clients in a group.

WEEKS 4 AND 5: AS THE WORLD TURNS

I described in my last log a very difficult group session with 28 clients where I was unable to foster involvement by any more than a handful of them, thus failing to fulfill the goals of my GAS. My solution was to restructure the group called "World." The therapist who I am covering for told me that the goal of the group is client involvement, and that I can use any means to achieve it.

What I did was to number 28 cards and write in different colored markers two words on each, on the first a category, i.e., "fruit," and on the bottom the specific item, i.e., "papaya." I sat the clients in a circle and gave out the cards at random. Then, the client with card

#1 asked the client with card #2 the category. Then the client with card #2 had to guess the specific category and if they couldn't then the whole group would join in guessing. Then the client with #2 asked #3, so that everyone asked a question and answered a question, and the group as a whole listened and helped. It worked. Nobody slept. They had a great time, and the struggle was to prevent the group answering before the person whose turn it was had given up. Many clients at the end told us they enjoyed it.

WE THE PEOPLE

The next week, week 5, my therapist asked me to do something on the Constitution and gave me a copy to read. I was at a total loss as to how to inspire interest in so dry a document. So anticipating the fall elections, what I did was to stage Presidential elections with myself and Bean Bomrind (the other occupational therapy student) as the candidates. In the format of a Town Meeting, the clients asked us our opinion on various topics of their choice, such as drugs, crime, abortion, and gave their opinions too. It was very lively, and particularly interesting was how clients reacted to a female presidential candidate. Although most (10 out of 19) clients participated actively by speaking up, and the group "glowed," I feel I should have thought of a format that could have forced more clients to participate, much as had happened the previous week. However, if voting for us is included as participation then the results were better. They nearly all voted. (I won.)

I would say so much more because I run a crafts group, too, where we did a leather-lacing (change purse) project, where I encouraged people to discuss their feelings about doing the craft ("it relaxes me," "--- give it to my boyfriend," "it breaks my ---.") and some fascinating things come up at team meetings. But I will limit myself to saying that finally after five weeks in this Center, I heard delusional ideation and hallucination from clients, expressed without a trace of guile and with complete sincerity. One man was very upset and said that he couldn't lace because a queen bee flew through him (I think a reaction to being mildly stressed by his therapist), and another man stated how hurtful it is for a 30 year old person to realize that he had been aborted as a fetus, and that young (child criminals) are really "controlled" when they do things. These are people I have gotten to know who never indicated such thought process before, and it shook me profoundly and made me realize just what they are struggling with.

WEEK 6: THE LAST WEEK

Our last week at F.E.G.S. was permeated with a feeling of reluctance to end what had become an enriching experience. Relationships had been established with clients, therapists and other students and it was hard to have to sever them.

Additionally, I felt that just as I was gaining insight into some of the clients, the process ended. One example is a client who spent 30 years in a state hospital, who rarely speaks and walks in fixed circles. His mouth hangs open, and if asked a question he may answer, but only after a long pause. Suddenly during group therapy he started to bellow aloud about punishing the person "who stole my mind away from me." When he had calmed down he related details from his communion as a boy, describing laurels around the door and vivid details as if he were there. I hadn't imagined his mind was working or that he possessed insight, and was very surprised to find otherwise. These types of reflection lead to narrative reasoning (Neistadt, 1996) which I feel can further lead to fruitful interactions for clients.

My crafts group took making banks out of coffee cans very seriously, decorating them with craft paper and patterned ribbons and bows. Even people who were pretty detached and out of it expressed marked preferences for different designs and colors, indicating that activity really brings out positive elements of personality that might otherwise remain submerged, just as M.O.H.O. describes. I had made friends with a drama therapy intern and asked to attend his group, a small one of five or six clients. He got them to express anger, to shout and act out. I wasn't sure that was such a good idea with chronic schizophrenics because I think it can unsettle them. I understand that his psychodynamic frame of reference encourages catharsis, but I think it should be used in a measured manner with goal direction, and that certain buried feelings are best left that way.

Anita, my supervisor, ran a large group where I taught some deaf clients a card game, "Concentration." I was beaten fair and square, and I liked how they interacted and helped each other out, applauding another participant's successes.

One drawback with using novel approaches to my "World" group was that it is difficult to use them twice. I had to devise a new format, and chose to give out cards with a question on it for that person to answer as they felt. Questions included: "What's the best thing to do when you feel lonely . . . or sad?" etc., or "What's the nicest thing you could do for another person?" Everyone received a card and spoke, and much useful advice was exchanged. I was gratified to end F.E.G.S. with a +1 on my GAS, but more gratified when a lady who had never done more than moan and snarl smiled sweetly and asked if she could please read her card, and then briefly answered it.

At the end of that session many people gathered around us to wish us well and thank us. It was an emotional experience because they were very sincere. Our therapist hoped that F.E.G.S. would start hiring occupational therapists and told us that if they do they might contact us!

LOG SUMMARY

The ratings below are the scores for the Psychomotor/Cognitive Goal Attainment Scale for the learning contract.

Sept.	17	crafts	− 1
	24	crafts	− 1
	25	creative writing	+1
	25	world	− 1
Oct.	1	crafts	+ 1
	2	world	+ 1
	8	crafts	+ 1
	9	world	0
	15	crafts	+ 1
	16	world	+ 2

I am fortunate to have chosen a goal which was very appropriate to the setting and population of the fieldwork placement, but which also tied in with my own needs for professional growth. The goal was to involve most of the participants in a group, and because schizophrenia seems to evoke a detachment and loss of touch with reality, involvement was a pertinent goal. For my part, not having had much experience with groups or a psychiatric population, I needed to acquire confidence in handling groups. That confidence was acquired not only because I had to, as my supervisor put it, "sink or swim," but in part because having set up a formal goal it became a challenge to achieve it, and the challenge outweighed the fear to the extent of almost eliminating fear.

Additionally, the effect of a focused goal was that I sought strategies to achieve it, and if I felt that a change in a group would further the goal, I made the change. This led to fluidity in group formats, and I am sure that without the goal I would not have deviated much from the set group protocol. Certainly there is much to be said for groups where the clients suggest the activity, but I noticed at my last "world" group that the more aware clients expressed curiosity and anticipation as to what we had "cooked up" for them this time. There was an interest and entertainment element of change planned by the student leaders that didn't really threaten them.

At the point when I could say that I was consistently achieving my goals I would have re-estimated and reformulated them, had the fieldwork continued. The next stage would have been to focus on the *quality* rather than the extent of client involvement.

The introduction of a frame of reference (M.O.H.O.) when assessing a client was useful in that I was compelled to assume a perspective which I normally would not arrive at, and so now I consider use of a frame of reference as a means to broaden rather than narrow the arsenal of strategies available for therapy.

Lyons' and Hayes' (1993) research regarding maintenance of social distance indicates that negative attitudes towards those with psychiatric difficulties are prevalent amongst occupational therapy students, to the degree that they are ranked 19 in a continuum of disabilities (with alcoholism and criminality as 20-21). At issue are beliefs and feelings rather than therapeutic skills, and amongst Lyons' solutions would be to engender contact beyond the clinical setting, socially and recreationally. His other two solutions, student reflection through a diary or log keeping and discussion (similar to our fieldwork seminars), and educational input from persons with psychiatric difficulties are in fact included in the S.U.N.Y., Health Science Center at Brooklyn curriculum. I must admit that my attitudes changed considerably during the course of fieldwork, but I feel it was primarily due to the elimination of the apprehension of being at risk and the friendliness and appreciation shown to me by the clients at F.E.G.S. Other students in the class had less gratifying experiences, so perhaps pleasant social interaction is a viable remedy to the problem.

Tryssenaar (1995) contends that although it is not possible to teach every skill for every practice area, teaching the skills of reflection can help meet that challenge. Presumably the theory is that versatility in the acquisition of therapeutic skills is made possible by reflection, which is summarized as "several complex skills leading towards the transformation of future action" (p. 696). Keeping a journal crystallized aspects of the fieldwork experience which I would otherwise not have noticed. Usually the gamut of emotions one encounters in new situations are incidental features, but as indicators of growth they can be useful. Positive feedback and "dialogue" which was offered by the course instructor's feedback was also very encouraging, as is the feeling that someone is taking an interest in one's progress. In addition, an interactive journal helps refocus goals, which can fade as the pressures of fieldwork assignments take over.

Confidence was the principle focus of the aspect of therapeutic self which was featured in my affective Goal Attainment Scale. I find it to be dependent on vision and preparation. I envision a situation, but don't envision myself managing it, and so feel that I am not confident, which affects performance. Being prepared even somewhat allows envisioning outcomes other than failure, and in fact when I went into a group session to lead it with a plan of action I thought would work, I felt confident.

Schwartz's (1984) occupational therapy student levels based on Loevinger's (1977) ego stages indicate a progression from reliance on a supervisor for attitudes and structure to the more independent status of achiever. My supervisor encouraged and aided us in our leading groups with minimal interference, and that combined with the need to quickly achieve proficiency enabled me to, I feel, become an achiever in some areas. I can only hope that my Level II fieldwork supervisors allow the same latitude to learn by experimentation with the inevitable failure/success ratio that accompanies it.

REFERENCES

Kielhofner, G. (1992). *Conceptual Foundations of Occupational Therapy.* Philadelphia: Davis.

Kiresuk, T., & Sherman, R. (1968). Goal attainment scaling: A general method of evaluating comprehensive mental health programs. *Community Mental Health Journal, 4,* 443-453.

Loevinger, J. (1977). *Ego Development: Conceptions and Theories.* San Francisco, CA: Jossey-Bass, 1977.

Lyons, M., & Hayes, R. (1993). Student perceptions of persons with psychiatric and other disorders. *American Journal of Occupational Therapy, 47*(6), 541-548.

Neistadt, M.E. (1996). Teaching strategies for the development of clinical reasoning. *American Journal of Occupational Therapy, 50*(8), 676-684.

Ottenbacher, K. J. & Cusick, A. (1990). Goal attainment scaling as a method of clinical service evaluation. *American Journal of Occupational Therapy, 44* (6), 676-684

Schwartz, K.R. (1984). An approach to supervision of students on fieldwork. *American Journal of Occupational Therapy, 38*(6), 393-397.

Scott, A. H. (1998). Learning contracts and the use of goal attainment scaling (GAS) for occupational therapy students on mental health fieldwork: An integrated approach to fieldwork learning. *Occupational Therapy in Mental Health, 14* (1/2), 119-127.

Scott, A. H. & Haggerty, E. J. (1984). Structuring goals via goal attainment scaling in occupational therapy groups in a partial hospitalization setting. *Occupational Therapy in Mental Health, 4*(2), 39-58.

Tryssenaar, J. (1995). Interactive journals: An educational strategy to promote reflection. *American Journal of Occupational Therapy, 49*(7), 695-702.

Index

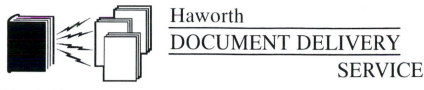

Haworth
DOCUMENT DELIVERY
SERVICE

This valuable service provides a single-article order form for any article from a Haworth journal.

- *Time Saving:* No running around from library to library to find a specific article.
- *Cost Effective:* All costs are kept down to a minimum.
- *Fast Delivery:* Choose from several options, including same-day FAX.
- *No Copyright Hassles:* You will be supplied by the original publisher.
- *Easy Payment:* Choose from several easy payment methods.

Open Accounts Welcome for . . .
- Library Interlibrary Loan Departments
- Library Network/Consortia Wishing to Provide Single-Article Services
- Indexing/Abstracting Services with Single Article Provision Services
- Document Provision Brokers and Freelance Information Service Providers

---

MAIL or *FAX* THIS ENTIRE ORDER FORM TO:

Haworth Document Delivery Service
The Haworth Press, Inc.
10 Alice Street
Binghamton, NY 13904-1580

or FAX: 1-800-895-0582
or CALL: 1-800-429-6784
9am-5pm EST

PLEASE SEND ME PHOTOCOPIES OF THE FOLLOWING SINGLE ARTICLES:

1) Journal Title: _____

    Vol/Issue/Year: _____ Starting & Ending Pages: _____

Article Title: _____

2) Journal Title: _____

    Vol/Issue/Year: _____ Starting & Ending Pages: _____

Article Title: _____

3) Journal Title: _____

    Vol/Issue/Year: _____ Starting & Ending Pages: _____

Article Title: _____

4) Journal Title: _____

    Vol/Issue/Year: _____ Starting & Ending Pages: _____

Article Title: _____

(See other side for Costs and Payment Information)

COSTS: Please figure your cost to order quality copies of an article.

1. Set-up charge per article: $8.00
   ($8.00 × number of separate articles)   _____

2. Photocopying charge for each article:
   1-10 pages: $1.00   _____

   11-19 pages: $3.00   _____

   20-29 pages: $5.00   _____

   30+ pages: $2.00/10 pages   _____

3. Flexicover (optional): $2.00/article   _____

4. Postage & Handling: US: $1.00 for the first article/
   $.50 each additional article   _____

   Federal Express: $25.00   _____

   Outside US: $2.00 for first article/
   $.50 each additional article _____

5. Same-day FAX service: $.50 per page   _____

   GRAND TOTAL: _____

METHOD OF PAYMENT: (please check one)

❏ Check enclosed   ❏ Please ship and bill. PO # _____
   (sorry we can ship and bill to bookstores only! All others must pre-pay)

❏ Charge to my credit card: ❏ Visa;   ❏ MasterCard;   ❏ Discover;
   ❏ American Express;

Account Number:_____ Expiration date:_____

Signature: ✗ _____

Name: _____ Institution: _____

Address: _____

_____

City: _____ State:_____ Zip:_____

Phone Number: _____ FAX Number: _____

MAIL or *FAX* THIS ENTIRE ORDER FORM TO:

Haworth Document Delivery Service	**or FAX:** 1-800-895-0582
The Haworth Press, Inc.	**or CALL:** 1-800-429-6784
10 Alice Street	(9am-5pm EST)
Binghamton, NY 13904-1580	